ONE MEAL A DAY INTERMITTENT FASTING

HOW TO LOSE WEIGHT EFFORTLESSLY, IMPROVE YOUR HEALTH, INCREASE MENTAL CLARITY, ACTIVATE AUTOPHAGY, AND HAVE MORE ENERGY

KATE MCCARTHY

© **Copyright 2020 Kate McCarthy - All rights reserved.**

The content contained within this book may not be reproduced, duplicated or transmitted without direct written permission from the author or the publisher.

Under no circumstances will any blame or legal responsibility be held against the publisher, or author, for any damages, reparation, or monetary loss due to the information contained within this book, either directly or indirectly.

Legal Notice:

This book is copyright protected. It is only for personal use. You cannot amend, distribute, sell, use, quote or paraphrase any part, or the content within this book, without the consent of the author or publisher.

Disclaimer Notice:

Please note the information contained within this document is for educational and entertainment purposes only. All effort has been executed to present accurate, up to date, reliable, complete information. No warranties of any kind are declared or implied. Readers acknowledge that the author is not engaged in the rendering of legal, financial, medical or professional advice. The content within this book has been derived from various sources. Please consult a licensed professional before attempting any techniques outlined in this book.

By reading this document, the reader agrees that under no circumstances is the author responsible for any losses, direct or indirect, that are incurred as a result of the use of the information contained within this document, including, but not limited to, errors, omissions, or inaccuracies.

DOWNLOAD YOUR FREE CHEAT SHEET

(Don't start fasting before you've consulted this cheat sheet...)

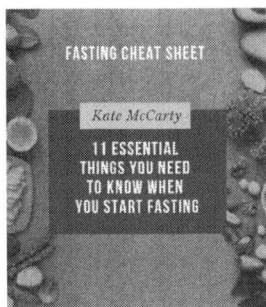

This cheat sheet includes:

- 11 things to know and to do while you are fasting.
- Why you need to know those things to start successfully.
- These things will make the process easier and more enjoyable.

The last thing I want is that the fasting process will be uncomfortable.

To receive your fasting cheat sheet, scan this QR code:

CONTENTS

Introduction: The Intermittent Fasting Trend   vii

1. Your Body on Intermittent Fasting   1
2. The Many Health Benefits of Intermittent Fasting   19
3. The Most Popular Ways to Do Intermittent Fasting   43
4. One Meal A Day Method of Intermittent Fasting   63
5. Preparing to Follow the OMAD Method of Intermittent Fasting   83
6. The Potential Risks and Side Effects of the OMAD Method   119

Conclusion: Your Intermittent Fasting Journey   137
References   143

INTRODUCTION: THE INTERMITTENT FASTING TREND

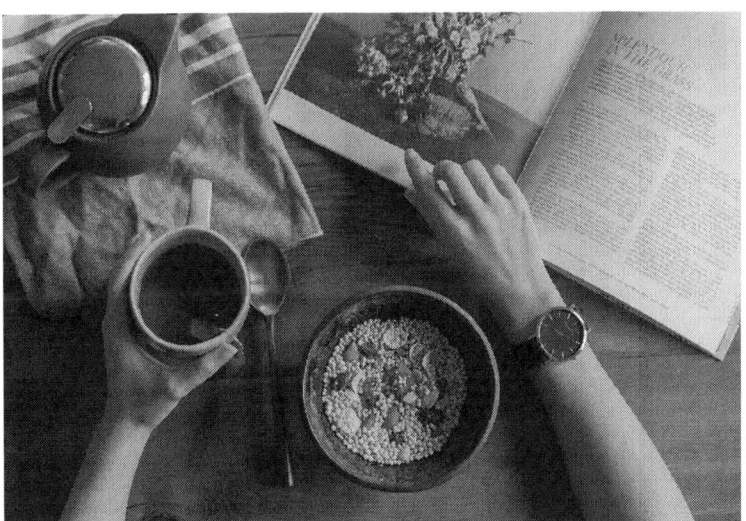

Fig. 1: IF. Pixabay, by The 5th, 2016, https://pixabay.com/photos/breakfast-healthy-food-diet-fruit-1663295/ Copyright 2016 by The 5th/Pixabay.

> "Fasting is the first principle of medicine; fast and see the strength of the spirit reveal itself."
>
> — RUMI

Are you tired of the endless diets you have been following that don't seem to be doing anything to improve your health? Or are you interested in making a significant change in your diet, and you're looking for the best option out there?

No matter what your reasons are for picking up this book, you're about to learn a lot of interesting information that can change your life for the better. You may have already heard about the intermittent fasting trend. After all, people all over the world are following intermittent fasting or "IF" and raving about how great their journeys are since they followed this eating pattern. The fact is, intermittent fasting isn't a diet—it's more of an eating pattern or lifestyle that comes with its own rules and guidelines.

If you're interested in learning about IF, specifically about the One Meal A Day (OMAD) method, then you have just chosen the best book for your health journey. Intermittent fasting is a powerful eating pattern that provides so many health benefits when followed correctly. Physiologically speaking, when you restrict your caloric intake by fasting intermittently, this can help increase your lifespan while improving your resistance to several metabolic factors that cause stress to the body (Hine, et. al., 2014). Evidence of this has been seen in studies conducted on animals, although more research is needed on humans to solidify this fact. However, those who support intermittent fasting believe that it can cause a special kind of immune response that repairs the cells of the body while stimulating several positive metabolic changes too.

Another essential benefit of intermittent fasting is weight-loss. This also happens to be one of the most common reasons why people decide to follow IF. Although other methods of fasting aren't associated with sustainable weight loss results, intermittent fasting works differently. As you follow this eating pattern, it gives your body an automatic caloric deficit, thus, promoting the burning of fat in your body. It also boosts your metabolism in the process and prevents you from getting cravings during your fasting windows. According to research, it promotes fat loss instead of water weight or muscle mass compared to dietary detoxes, cleanses, or extremely low-calorie diets. In fact, one review has shown that IF can help you lose up to 7% of your waist circumference in less than two months (Barnosky, et. al., 2014). This means that fat loss occurs in the belly, which is very beneficial as belly fat can cause harm to your organs.

These are just some of the benefits you can look forward to when you start intermittent fasting. There are many more that we will be discussing later. One thing I can tell you right now is that intermittent fasting isn't a strict eating pattern that will make you feel deprived. There are different methods for following IF and you can choose the best way to suit your lifestyle. Because of this flexibility, the technique that makes the most sense to you can be your new method for eating throughout the day.

Typically, intermittent fasting involves alternate periods of eating (feeding windows) with periods of fasting (fasting windows). While fasting, you wouldn't consume any solids, but you can have non-caloric beverages like water, tea, and coffee. Sometimes, you can even have a bowl of broth if you're feeling really hungry. When it comes to IF, you don't focus on restricting or eliminating certain foods from your diet. Instead, you would focus more on your eating schedule. But before we go any further, let me share my story and how intermittent fasting has changed my life. Hopefully, this can inspire you to keep reading so that you can learn everything about this eating pattern and how it can change your life for the better too.

When I was in my early 20s, I started suffering from insulin resistance. Since I was so young, this came as a shock to me. This condition increased my risk of developing diabetes, and it also affected my weight. Although I wasn't particularly health-conscious before getting diagnosed with insulin resistance, I was pretty confident about my diet and health habits. Despite this, I had to start taking medications to prevent my condition from getting worse. However, regardless of the medicinal and

INTRODUCTION: THE INTERMITTENT FASTING TREND | xi

diet interventions I had, my insulin sensitivity didn't improve enough for me to get my previous life back. Knowing this was very hard for me. At such a young age, I already had a condition that I felt would ruin the rest of my life.

Instead of giving up, I decided to make healthier life choices. Since medications weren't helping me in the big way that I thought they would, I started researching holistic and alternative practices when I turned 30. By then, I was already suffering for years, both physically and psychologically. I knew that I had to do something to make things better so that I wouldn't experience depression. Through my research, I had come across intermittent fasting. At the time, it was one of the emerging trends in the diet world, and from the first time I had read about it, I was hooked.

In particular, I was very interested in the One Meal A Day approach, otherwise known as OMAD. As a person who leads a hectic and unpredictable lifestyle, the OMAD method of intermittent fasting seemed very interesting to me. I felt like it would fit my routine perfectly. Of course, the OMAD method was very different from my then-current eating habits. Through my research, I knew that forcing myself to follow this method right away would cause more problems for me, healthwise.

Since I had never tried fasting before, I took things slowly. I learned all the methods of IF and how to do them. Then I chose the most basic method and started incorporating it into my routine. It was definitely a change for me, and I did experience all of the things I had read about. To make things easier, I focused on choosing the right foods to eat during my feeding windows to ensure that I was getting all the nutrients my body needed to stay healthy. I also started practicing meditation and mindfulness, which made the journey easier too. I had the determination to commit to this eating pattern and after some time, I saw concrete results. Amazingly, I was able to lose a total of 50 pounds from the weight I gained because of my insulin resistance!

Apart from this, my doctors also told me that my condition had improved so much since I started IF that they gave me the go-signal to stop taking medications! This piece of news made me over-the-moon happy. It also inspired me to write this book and another one about Water Fasting, another highly effective method that has helped me achieve my health and diet goals. Whether you are experiencing the same situation I experienced, or you just want to make positive changes in your life, I hope this book can help you out. Here, I summed up everything I learned when I researched about intermittent fasting and the OMAD method.

As someone who has suffered through a medical condition that changed my life drastically, I wrote this book with compassion and love. Throughout my journey, I received no less from my friends and family, so now, I want to pay it forward by helping others get through their struggles. No matter what your struggles are right now, I hope that this book will help transform your life for the better. By learning about IF here, I hope that you can start following this amazing eating pattern so that you can experience the health improvements that are hidden in such simple practices.

1

YOUR BODY ON INTERMITTENT FASTING

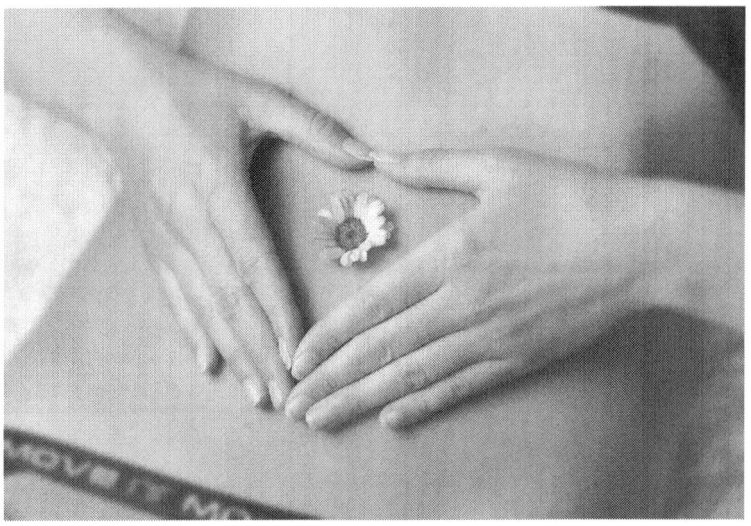

Fig. 2: Healthy Body. Pixabay, by silviarita, 2018, https://pixabay. com/photos/belly-heart-love-girl-relaxation-3186730/ Copyright 2018 by silviarita/Pixabay.

Intermittent fasting is a unique eating pattern that can potentially benefit your health in different ways. In fact, there are so many research studies conducted on IF and its effects, and most of these show promising results. Usually, the animal subjects and even the human participants of these studies have experienced weight loss and an improvement in their cholesterol levels. Researchers found that it can even be used as part of the treatment for certain conditions. While most of these studies have been conducted on rats, almost all studies on humans have also shown that IF is both effective and safe. More importantly, choosing the right method of IF can make this eating pattern more effective, realistic, and sustainable for you to reach your health goals.

Although fasting has already been a concept since the dawn of time, recently, IF has become one of the more popular approaches for losing weight. Different forms of fasting have existed for ages, especially as a tool for weight loss. But in the year 2012, Dr. Michael Mosley, a broadcast journalist of BBC, had popularized intermittent fasting in his TV documentary entitled, "Eat Fast, Live Longer," and his book, "The Fast Diet." After these came out—and gained public interest—a journalist by the name of Kate Harrison launched her own book entitled, "The 5:2 Diet," which was based on her own experiences. Subsequently, Dr. Jason Fung, a nephrologist from Canada, came out with his own bestselling book in 2016 entitled, "The Obesity Code." Soon, intermittent fasting received a constant stream of positive buzz as more and more people started following it and experienced the benefits. Then these people started sharing their stories, which, in turn, helped IF explode in popularity in such a short time.

Before you start following this eating pattern, learning everything that you can about it will help you out immensely. Understanding the science behind IF may help you understand why it works so well. This understanding also makes it easier for you to believe other people when they share their own experiences with IF, whether good or bad. So, in this book, I have combined my own anecdotal experiences along with the stories shared by others I know, plus all of the research I had conducted as I embarked on my own IF journey. To give you a clear picture of what IF is all about and what it does to your body, I will share some of the studies I have read plus sensible advice on nutrition to provide you with everything you need to start fasting intermittently.

When you read about IF, you might think that it's too hard for you to follow. But the truth is, it doesn't have to be. One of the best things about intermittent fasting is that there are many ways to do it. For instance, if you try fasting on alternate days, you may experience the same benefits as trying to fast at specific times each day. If you have never tried fasting before, then fasting for an entire day might be too challenging for you. That's okay because you can ease into IF until you feel more confident about trying the more extreme methods of this eating pattern.

When it comes to following IF, you may have to try different methods before finding the one that is most effective for you. The method you choose should fit your lifestyle, and it must be sustainable for you. Combine this with a healthy diet, and you're sure to find success with intermittent fasting. On the other hand, if you only consume processed or junk foods on IF, you will place yourself at risk for the common dangers and side effects of this diet. This is where the value of research comes in. The more you learn about IF, the more you can prepare yourself for what is to come. Also, you won't have to panic when you start experiencing changes in your body because of the new eating pattern that you follow.

Personally, I do believe in intermittent fasting. In particular, I am a follower of the One Meal A Day or OMAD method. This is one of the more extreme ways, but I didn't start with it right away. My intermittent fasting journey involved trying out different methods until I found the right one. That was when I experienced the benefits that this trendy eating pattern had to offer. Unfortunately, when it comes to OMAD, there aren't a lot of resources that provide comprehensive information about it. I had to do a lot of research just to understand this method, how to follow it correctly, and even the potential risks it comes with. The good news is, after discussing the basics of intermittent fasting, we will be focusing on the

OMAD method to help you determine if it is the right one for you.

WHAT IS INTERMITTENT FASTING?

If you're thinking about the best ways to improve your health, then intermittent fasting might help you out. Intermittent fasting isn't a diet—it's an eating pattern wherein you would cycle between eating and fasting. While diets focus on the quantity and quality of the food you eat, intermittent fasting focuses on when you eat or the timing. This is why the main difference between the various methods of intermittent fasting is the variation in schedules. Later, we will discuss these methods in detail.

As you follow intermittent fasting, you would have "feasting windows" and "fasting windows." During your feasting windows, you allow yourself to eat whatever you want for a certain period of time. Usually, this would last for a specific number of hours. Then when your fasting window starts, you would stop consuming solid foods or beverages that contain calories. However, you can consume non-caloric beverages like water or plain tea and coffee.

If you fast long enough, your insulin levels will go down to the point where your body switches from burning glucose to burning fat. At this point, your body reaches a metabolic state known as "ketosis" wherein it becomes a fat-burning machine.

Another way to look at it is this: when you fast long enough, you starve your body of glucose, its primary source of energy. As soon as your body's glucose stores have been depleted, ketosis kicks in. Then your body turns to your fat stores to keep it functioning. But fat-burning isn't the only benefit of ketosis. In the same way, intermittent fasting also offers a number of health benefits, which we will go through in the next chapter.

While intermittent fasting is a relatively new concept in the sense that it is now being used for weight loss and other health purposes, the actual practice of fasting has been around from the beginning. Many religions and cultures have been fasting as part of their ancient traditions. For instance, Theravada Buddhist monks practice fasting as part of their monastic training. From noon to the time the sun rises on the next day, they practice fasting—and they do this every day. Islam also practices fasting, using a method similar to IF during Ramadan. In the morning, before dawn, they consume a meal to prepare themselves for the fast. From dawn until the sun sets, they don't eat anything. Then in the evening, they allow themselves to eat again. However, they only do this for one month, and it's not part of their normal lifestyle. These are just two of the most common examples of how fasting is utilized as a part of religious practices.

Apart from this, fasting has also been used in a therapeutic way at least since the year 1915. Back then, it was used to help treat people who suffered from obesity. Around the 1960s, the medical community had a renewed interest in fasting. This time, they focused on short-term or intermittent fasts to determine the health benefits these fasts have to offer. Since then, intermittent scientists and researchers have conducted so many studies about IF that when 2012 rolled in, this eating pattern suddenly became all the rage.

Intermittent fasting will only work if you follow it correctly. No matter what method you have chosen, it's essential for you to fast completely during your fasting window. This means no snacks whatsoever, not even a sugary drink with whipped cream on top. If this is your first time fasting, then IF might be a challenge for you. However, the longer you stick with the eating pattern, the more your body will adjust to it. When this happens, then you will find it easier to follow IF. Unlike diets, you won't have to restrict yourself from eating certain foods or eliminate specific food groups from your diet. Of course, it would still be more beneficial for you if you focus on whole foods to ensure that you are getting all the nutrients you need to keep your body healthy.

One factor that would contribute to which method of IF you choose is what your main purpose for following this eating pattern is. Take fat burning, for instance. This is one of the most common reasons why people decide to IF. This also happens to be one of my own reasons for fasting intermittently. To achieve the fat-burning benefit of intermittent fasting, your fasting windows should at least be 12 hours. Then if you can go higher than that, your body may become even more efficient at burning fat. Of course, as a beginner, you would have to work your way up to a fasting window as long as this.

Unlike other diets, fasting doesn't require you to count calories either. It's not a requirement, but it can be beneficial, especially if you want to avoid any health issues like nutrient deficiencies. Take me, for instance, since I follow the OMAD method, I found it more comforting to count the calories of my single meal for the day, especially when I was starting out. After all, I was trying to overcome my insulin resistance, so I made sure that I was doing everything right. Of course, if calorie counting isn't something that you want to do, you don't have to in order to follow IF correctly.

While many of us have found success with IF, this doesn't mean that it's for everyone. Some people have tried following IF but have found it too challenging to sustain. Others have tried too much too fast, which caused them to feel too much pressure. Then there are others who gave up because they didn't see the results or experience the benefits right away. At the end of the day, your success on IF will depend on how committed you are to follow it, how well it can fit into your lifestyle, and if you can follow the method you have chosen correctly. This means that you can only truly determine if intermittent fasting is right for you by trying it out after you have learned all that you can about it.

WHAT HAPPENS TO YOUR BODY WHEN YOU EAT?

Before we discuss what happens to your body while fasting, let me help you understand what happens to your body whenever you eat. In a nutshell, this is what happens: right after eating something, your body starts producing insulin to convert the sugar in the food you ate, the sugar is used to fuel your cells, and whatever is left gets stored in your body as fat. However, these processes won't get triggered when you are following intermittent fasting. Instead, it will result in the activation of other bodily mechanisms.

After eating a meal, the process of digestion follows naturally. Digestion is a process that involves the conversion of food into fuel for the body to absorb and utilize for energy. Digestion can also convert the food you have eaten into raw materials for building or repairing tissues. From head to toe, all of the parts of your body require this energy to keep functioning. All of the organs and systems in your body need fuel to keep functioning. When you eat regularly, the food you eat is the primary energy source of your body.

The digestion process also involves the production of enzymes and acids that mix with the food you eat to break everything down. During this process, the carbohydrate content of your food—the starches and sugars—are broken down into glucose. Then your small intestines and stomach absorb this glucose before releasing it into your bloodstream. After that, the glucose can already be used for energy as needed while any leftover is stored for later use. For your body to start using or storing glucose, it needs the hormone insulin. Without this hormone, glucose remains in your bloodstream, which, in turn, keeps your levels of blood sugar elevated.

The pancreas is the organ in your body that produces insulin. This organ contains beta cells that are highly sensitive to the glucose content in your bloodstream. These beta cells also check your blood glucose levels every couple of seconds so that they can determine whether they need to slow down or speed up the amount of insulin they produce and release. Whenever you eat a high-carb meal, your blood glucose level increases, thus, causing the beta cells in the pancreas to produce and release high amounts of insulin, allowing your body to use or store glucose. After this, your blood glucose levels will start decreasing, thus, causing the beta cells in the pancreas to slow down insulin production.

Throughout the day (and night), this process occurs. The beta cells in your pancreas check your blood glucose regularly. If you are healthy, then your pancreas and beta cells will work normally. The process of utilizing energy and keeping a delicate balance with just the right amount of insulin from the pancreas is essential for your body to maintain the energy it needs to function even while you sleep. However, if you suffer from insulin resistance, this throws your hormone levels off, thus, leading to other issues inside your body. Or if you keep eating throughout the day, especially if you love eating high-carb foods, your body would always need high amounts of insulin. Eventually, your body might not have the capacity to keep up with the amount of food coming in, and your bodily functions start breaking down.

This is where fasting comes in. When you fast, you are giving your body, specifically your digestive system, time to rest, and recuperate. Also, when you don't consume anything, the beta cells in your pancreas won't have to produce insulin since there won't be spikes in your blood glucose levels. Since intermittent fasting involves cycling between periods of eating and fasting, this means that you won't be starving yourself completely. You will eat at some point, but you will be reducing the frequency of your meals so that your body can work more efficiently.

WHAT HAPPENS TO YOUR BODY WHEN YOU FAST INTERMITTENTLY?

Fasting means that you wouldn't consume anything with calories. It's crucial for you to understand the "no calories" part, especially when you start following IF. Just because you're allowed to drink during your fasting windows, this doesn't mean that you can whip up smoothies or blended drinks when you are hungry. Drinking such beverages would break your fast because the sugars and all other calories in these drinks will activate your body's digestive process. If you have been "fasting" this way and you haven't experienced any benefits, those sugary and high-calorie drinks are to blame.

Anyway, going back to fasting... when you stop eating for hours at a time, your body will start working differently. In a nutshell, here are the things that will happen:

- After your body digests the last bit of food from the last meal you ate, it won't be breaking down anything else. Therefore, glucose won't be released into your bloodstream, which, in turn, signals the pancreas to stop producing insulin.
- When there is no more glucose to use, this is when your body turns to the fat stores in your cells for energy.
- With the absence of glucose and insulin, your blood sugar levels stabilize. You won't experience spikes or crashes that tend to make you feel tired or sometimes make you crave certain types of food.
- The longer you fast, the more efficient your body becomes in terms of using energy. This won't happen if you fast intermittently for a week. You may start seeing the benefits if you continue following IF regularly for a couple of months. In the beginning, you may feel tired and have a lack of focus. But when your body starts adjusting, your energy levels will go back up, thus, making you feel better.
- Fasting also gives your digestive system and gut a

much-needed break. It provides a chance to slow down and reset, which, in turn, promotes improvements in the body like a reduction of acid reflux, heartburn, bloating, and other common issues.

As you can see, intermittent fasting works by helping your body learn how to work in a different way. Because of the flexibility of IF, it has become one of the most popular diet trends in the world now. As long as you follow the method or schedule you have chosen consistently and adequately; you can expect to see the benefits of this eating pattern happening after some time.

However, simple as this eating pattern is, it may throw your body "out of whack," especially during the first few days or weeks of your IF journey. This is especially true if you haven't tried fasting before or if you usually eat heavy meals or frequent snacks throughout the day. In such cases, starting on IF means that you would be significantly restricting your food intake. This means that you will feel hungry, and you may experience a number of weird side effects. These are normal... I have experienced some of these too. The important thing is to stick with the eating pattern so that you can give your body time to adjust to it.

Even our earliest ancestors practiced intermittent fasting, although they didn't have a name for it back then. In the past, our ancestors didn't have access to readily-available foods. Therefore, they would only eat when they felt hungry, and before they could eat, they would have to hunt or forage first. If they couldn't find anything, they would be forced to fast. These fasts depended on where and when they would find their next meal. This shows us that back then, snacking wasn't part of their lifestyle. It has only become an extra part of our daily diet since food has become so abundant and readily available to us. Unfortunately, snacking isn't a healthy habit, and it's a definite no-no when you are fasting.

Fasting affects your body in the same way exercise does. When you exercise, your cells experience some level of stress. However, during your workout, those cells don't grow or strengthen—these things happen during the resting or recovery period. In the same way, your cells enter a stress-resistance mode while you fast. It super-charges them so that when you start eating again, they can quickly absorb the nutrients you consume, thus, allowing them to grow and become stronger. This is another way for you to look at how fasting affects your body.

When you start fasting, expect to experience hunger. No matter what method you choose to follow, hunger pangs are one of the most common side effects you will feel, especially when you start fasting intermittently. This is because your body is used to getting a steady supply of glucose from the foods you eat. During your fasting window, your body will feel deprived, which, in turn, causes it to send specific signals that cause hunger pangs. Among all of the side effects you may experience, this is one of the most challenging to deal with. If you focus on your hunger pangs, you won't be able to think of anything else. This, of course, may lead you to convince yourself that it's okay to "just eat something light."

As much as possible, try to resist the urge to give in to your hunger pangs. There are many ways to do this, which we will discuss later. When you stick with your fasting window, your body will adjust to the habit of fasting. This is when your body will learn to use the fat stores in your body for fuel. The longer you remain in your fasting window, the more efficient your body gets at burning fat. Soon, you will notice that your hunger pangs don't happen as frequently as they did in the past. Your appetite will start leveling out, and you will have fewer cravings too.

However, if you feel that, at some point, your hunger pangs are starting to interfere with your life, then you may allow yourself to grab a quick bite. It's never a good idea to restrict yourself so much that you cannot think of anything else. The same thing goes if you start feeling dizzy or lightheaded during your fasting window. Your goal here isn't to starve yourself—it's to train your body to get used to eating less frequently each day. If you can do this without forcing yourself or making yourself feel bad, then you know that you are on the right path.

Now that you know what happens inside your body during your fasting window, you should have a better idea of what to expect when you start on your IF journey. Of course, there are things you can do to make the adjustment more comfortable and ensure your own health and safety. One of the most important things you can do to become successful at IF is to learn how to eat healthily. Although this isn't a requirement while following the eating pattern, it will help you achieve your health goals faster while avoiding the potential pitfalls and risks of IF.

Let's have a moment of reflection here. Try to think of yourself following the intermittent fasting eating pattern right now. Now, imagine that you have chosen to practice the OMAD method after a few months of following one of the easier IF methods. Each day, you would only eat one meal, and this meal would have to keep you full, satisfied, and nourished until the next day. With this in your mind, what kind of meal would you imagine yourself eating? Should it be something quick that you bought from a favorite fast food joint, or should it be something nutrient-dense that you prepared yourself? Should it be a fast-food burger with fries, fried chicken, and a milkshake or a full platter of colorful vegetables, meat, a bowl of soup, and a glass of fresh fruit juice? Between these two options, which do you think will make you feel full and nourished? When you start following IF, you can conduct your own experiments in terms of the food you will eat during your feasting window. This is the best way for you to really experience what will make you feel good and what won't.

As a concept, intermittent fasting has been around since the beginning. As you learn about fasting and its effects on your body, this will, hopefully, make the process less intimidating. After all, you are already fasting right now. From the time you have your last meal of the day to the time you have your first meal of the next day, this is already considered a fasting window. So you can actually plan your fasting window to include this time. It's all about coming up with the best strategy for your body to adjust, especially at the beginning.

IS INTERMITTENT FASTING RIGHT FOR YOU?

What is your main reason for wanting to follow intermittent fasting?

These days, most people give intermittent fasting a try because they want to lose weight. If this is your main reason or one of your reasons, then there is a very high possibility that intermittent fasting can help you out. However, as you may have already realized, IF offers more than just weight loss. This fantastic eating pattern can contribute to the actual improvement of your health, especially if you practice it correctly.

But how do you know that IF is right for you? Well, the best way to find out is to give it a try. In this chapter, you learned what intermittent fasting is and how it affects the body compared to when you eat consistently throughout the day. Of course, all of these things are just explanations to help you understand IF and prepare yourself for what to expect when you start it. Hopefully, everything you have discovered in this chapter has piqued your interest in the diet. Now, all you have to do is to keep exploring the different chapters. In each chapter, you will learn something new about IF until you reach a profound understanding of how you can use it to change your life.

In the pages of this book, I have also shared some of the most effective and practical tips to follow IF that I swear by. Since I started my IF journey with the purpose of overcoming my insulin resistance, I was driven to make it work. I committed to IF, and I learned everything I can to know exactly how I can follow this eating pattern and experience all the benefits it has to offer. You can learn this too and, hopefully, improve your health and your life as much as I have. At this point, the best advice I can give you is to keep moving forward. There is a reason why IF has surged in popularity and gained so many enthusiastic followers. And by learning all about it through this book, you can start your own IF journey and look forward to all the good things it can bring to your life. So, let's keep going!

2

THE MANY HEALTH BENEFITS OF INTERMITTENT FASTING

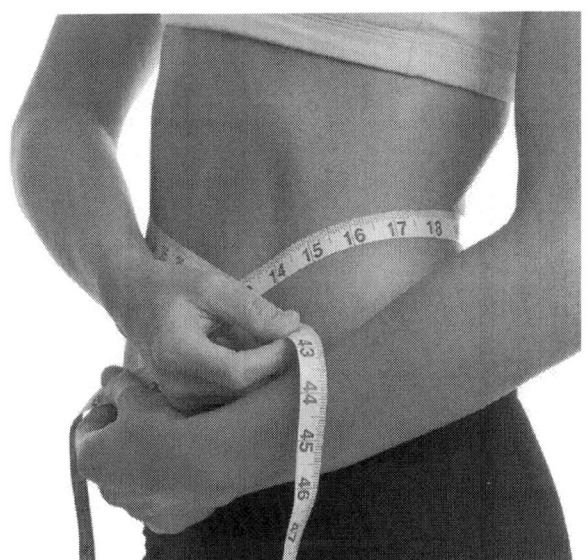

Fig. 3: Benefits. Unsplash, by Bill Oxford, 2019, https://unsplash.com/photos/aIlAhLdwk2g/ Copyright 2019 by Bill Oxford/Unsplash.

According to studies, both animal and human, intermittent fasting offers wide-ranging health benefits. Although more research is needed to solidify all of these claims, the sheer number of anecdotal reports and scientific evidence is already overwhelming enough to encourage people to believe in the potential of this eating pattern. And the fact that fasting has been around for centuries also strengthens the argument for IF, don't you think?

As someone who has done a lot of research on IF and has been following it for a long time now, I can attest to the benefits it has to offer. However, anecdotal reports shouldn't be enough for you. It's also helpful to read the studies and research conducted about IF to help you understand why these benefits exist and why they might not happen for you. This becomes even more important if you want to understand the scientific aspect of the benefits IF has to offer. Therefore, this chapter is dedicated to the benefits of intermittent fasting.

Here, I will share with you the good things that this eating pattern has to offer. I have included some of the most interesting studies I've read through research for you to have a deeper understanding of why this eating pattern changes the way your body works to promote the improvement of your health. Of course, you can also do your own research as you learn about IF. Just make sure that the resources you read offer truthful information. Sadly, there are many sites and written resources that tend to exaggerate the benefits without sharing the other side of the story. Intermittent fasting has a lot of potential benefits, but it also comes with its own risks. Finding out the good and bad sides of IF gives you a better look at the big picture. Later, we will be going through the potential risks to look out for. But for now, let's focus on the scientific and clinical side of the benefits intermittent fasting has to offer.

WEIGHT LOSS

Weight loss is an important benefit of intermittent fasting, although this isn't the only good thing that can come from following this eating plan. Since this is the most common benefit most people look forward to, let's discuss it first. One of the main problems with following a diet is sustainability. In the beginning, you may feel excited and motivated to follow a diet correctly, especially if you start seeing yourself lose weight. But when you get bored of the diet, you become too busy to follow it correctly, or you feel like it has become too challenging (because of the restrictions), then you might go back to your old diet. Often, this may result in regaining all of the weight you lost while on the diet. This is one of the main reasons why a lot of people jump from one diet to another.

This isn't something you would have to worry about with intermittent fasting. Since IF is an eating pattern, you can make it part of your lifestyle. One of the studies I have read confirmed that many people who decide to follow IF do so for the weight loss benefit (Johnstone, 2015). Since you won't be eating throughout the day as you might have been doing in the past IF will reduce the number of meals you eat each day. Furthermore, IF also enhances the functions of your hormones to promote weight loss. Of course, this would only apply if you eat normally during your feeding windows. You don't have to compensate for the meals you've missed by overeating at every meal. If you do this, then weight loss won't be one of the benefits you can expect from IF.

According to a review of the scientific literature of IF, it can cause a person to lose up to 8% of their overall weight over 3 to 24 weeks (Barnosky, et. al., 2014). During fasting, your insulin levels go down while norepinephrine and growth hormone levels go up. These hormonal changes promote fat burning for the body to have fuel to use for energy. Moreover, intermittent fasting can increase your metabolic rate by up to 14% to help your body burn more calories. This means that IF is highly effective for weight loss because it works in two main ways: it reduces your caloric intake and gives your metabolic rate a boost. In the same review conducted in 2014, IF helped the participants lose between 4% to 7% of the circumference of their waists. This means that a lot of the weight they lost came from their belly fat—where fat is typically stored.

Continuing on the topic of weight loss, another great thing about intermittent fasting is that it doesn't cause a lot of muscle loss compared to following a diet where you would have to restrict your caloric intake continuously. In one particular study, the results showed that IF only resulted in 10% muscle loss out of the total weight loss of the participants. Conversely, diets that promote caloric restriction resulted in 25% muscle loss out of the total weight loss (Varady, 2011). The findings of this study suggest that the diets might be as effective as intermittent fasting in terms of weight loss, but you won't have to sacrifice your muscle mass by following IF.

Although there are several other studies that focus on the weight loss aspect of intermittent fasting, these are the simplest to understand, and they provide great explanations for why IF promotes sustainable weight loss. Since this is the most sought-after benefit of the eating pattern, there are factors you can focus on to improve your chances. These factors include your calorie intake, the quality of food that you consume, your consistency, and a lot of patience. These can also promote the other health benefits that IF has to offer.

SLOW DOWN THE AGING PROCESS

The next benefit of IF that I will share with you is the delay of the aging process. Because of the changes that occur inside your body when you fast, this can help prevent or delay the onset of age-related medical conditions too. All methods of intermittent fasting offer this benefit. What's better is that you can enjoy this benefit even if weight loss doesn't come right away. The slowing down of the aging process and the delay of age-related conditions occur because of a process known as "metabolic switching."

The researchers of one particular study discovered the role of this process when it gets activated through intermittent fasting (Anton, et. al., 2017). When you fast, you will starve your body of glucose, which it needs for fuel. Because of this, your body resorts to a different source of energy. When this happens, your liver starts breaking fatty acids down into ketones, which your body then uses for fuel. Since this process stops when your feeding window begins, the process of breaking down fats stops too. But the good news is, intermittent fasting enables metabolic switching wherein your body switches between ketones and glucose, the primary sources of fuel.

According to the researchers, metabolic switching activates a lasting cellular response, which, in turn, provides a protective effect to the body. Alternating between fuel sources through intermittent fasting helps to reduce inflammation, protects your body against the damages of oxidative stress, and boosts your metabolism. All of these are important to prevent the onset of age-related diseases and to keep your body young and healthy. The best part is, these benefits keep coming even after you have gone back to "eating normally."

In another study, the researchers focused on the role of nutrition in preventing age-related disorders (Descamps, et. al., 2005). The results of this study suggest that intermittent fasting can promote an antioxidant effect along with the reduction of oxidative stress that causes aging and the diseases related to it. In particular, the calorie restriction aspect of intermittent fasting is behind this benefit. The restriction of calories by reducing the number of meals you consume each day supports specific mechanisms that promote healthy aging, namely antioxidant effects, autophagy, the proliferation of cells, inflammation, and mitochondrial physiology. All of these mechanisms are related to each other, and they all contribute to the aging benefit of IF.

Naturally, when the aging process slows down, it also lowers the risk of age-related diseases. This, in turn, may even extend your lifespan. Studies conducted on rats have shown that a longer lifespan is another benefit of intermittent fasting. In one of these studies, it showed that IF enhances the survival of mature rats even if they have passed the age at which the growth of their body weight typically comes to a halt (Goodrick, et. al., 1983). In another study that still focused on rats, the researchers discovered that IF helps slow down the rate of aging (Sogawa & Kubo, 2000). The results showed that IF helped increase the maximum lifespan of the rats while inhibiting the development of several age-related conditions. In this study, the rats that followed intermittent fasting lived longer than the rats that were always fully-fed. This also applied to the rats on IF that were heavier than the ones eating throughout the day. Although these studies were conducted on rats, age-related benefits and longevity remain to be well-documented benefits of intermittent fasting.

SAFELY IMPROVE TYPE-2 DIABETES AND METABOLIC SYNDROME

The benefits of intermittent fasting just keep coming as it can also be a safe intervention for the treatment of type-2 diabetes and metabolic syndrome. This easily tolerable eating pattern can help improve these conditions when followed correctly. However, if you suffer from these conditions or any type of medical condition for that matter, it's best to consult with your doctor first. It's not recommended to make any changes to your eating habits without first asking for advice from your personal physician. Your doctor might even offer you valuable advice about how to start fasting intermittently.

Going back to this benefit, let's start with type-2 diabetes. The main feature of this chronic condition is high levels of blood sugar in the context of insulin resistance. Since intermittent fasting helps reduce insulin resistance (this is one benefit that I have experienced firsthand) and helps lower your levels of blood sugar, it can help protect you against this disease. In one study, IF improved the conditions of middle-aged men who suffered from type-2 diabetes (Furmli, et. al., 2017). In this study, the researchers noted that the participants lost weight, they got well enough to stop taking insulin, and they also reduced the oral medication they were taking. According to the researchers, medications might not be as effective for treating this condition as dietary changes are. But when you change your diet, you would be addressing the underlying cause of the condition.

Another study highlighted the benefits of insulin on the improvement of insulin resistance (Barnosky, et. al., 2014). The results of this study showed that the participants showed a significant reduction in their levels of blood sugar. The researchers observed that the fasting blood sugar of participants went down by as much as 6% while their fasting insulin levels went down by as much as 31%. In a different study, the researchers suggested that IF can be a tolerable and safe dietary intervention in patients who suffered from type-2 diabetes (Arnason, et. al., 2017). This effect happens as the eating pattern improves the fasting glucose levels and the bodyweight of the patients. Yet another study supported the same findings as the researchers discovered that IF can help with weight loss, reduce the risk of the disease, and even improve memory (Carter, et. al., 2018).

Unlike type-2 diabetes, metabolic syndrome isn't a single disease. It's an umbrella term used for several risk factors of severe medical conditions like heart disease, stroke, and even diabetes. A recent study focused on the potential role of intermittent fasting in the improvement of metabolic syndrome (Wilkinson, et. al., 2019). This relatively new study looked at the weight loss and health benefits of the eating pattern in rodents and people. The results of this study had shown very promising potential in terms of using intermittent fasting as a lifestyle intervention in the treatment of people suffering from metabolic syndrome. The weight loss benefit of IF can improve the condition, especially when paired with other lifestyle changes like exercise and stress management.

This study involved a rigorous clinical trial where the participants were given a 10-hour feeding window where they had the freedom to eat what they want and when they want. Most of the participants in this study were obese, and more than 80% of them were taking medications. With the conditions set by the researchers, the participants had complete control over their diet within this feeding window, and they even had the opportunity to set the feeding window based on their regular daily schedule. Because of this freedom, the participants felt good about the schedule. As they started following the IF schedule, they started sleeping better and discovered that they had more energy. This prompted them to keep going. The clinical trial ran for three months, and by the end of it, the participants had an average BMI reduction of 3% with a 3% reduction of visceral or abdominal fat. These and all other improvements helped reduce the risk factors of metabolic syndrome. Moreover, the participants were very much willing to continue with intermittent fasting because they felt that it was easy to follow.

SUPPORTS CARDIOVASCULAR HEALTH

Cardiovascular disease is one of the most common causes of death in the world, but just like metabolic syndrome, this isn't a single disease. Cardiovascular disease encompasses different diseases, including hypertension, heart failure, stroke, atrial fibrillation, and so on. There are many risk factors associated with cardiovascular disease. Fortunately, there is evidence that IF has a positive effect on cardiovascular health by stabilizing cholesterol levels, reducing blood pressure, and improving the other risk factors of cardiovascular disease.

One study I have read focused on the weight loss benefit of intermittent fasting for the benefit of cardiovascular health (Varady, et. al., 2009). In this study, the researchers aimed to lower the risk of cardiovascular disease in obese individuals through the eating pattern. The findings of their study showed that intermittent fasting is, indeed, a viable option for those who suffer from obesity to shed their excess pounds and decrease their risk of cardiovascular disease. Another study about cardiovascular health focused on the metabolic effects of intermittent fasting on people who suffer chronic conditions that may lead to cardiovascular disease (de Azevedo, et. al., 2012). The researchers of this study reported that IF has positive effects on the metabolic disturbances caused by chronic conditions, thus, making it an accessible and viable intervention for the improvement of cardiovascular health.

There is some speculation that IF can also change our gut microbiome. The human microbiome consists of collective microorganism genomes. According to experts, these microorganisms are highly dynamic and they go through cyclical fluctuations in terms of their composition each day (Zarrinpar, et. al., 2014). Because of the nature of intermittent fasting and how it changes our metabolism, it can also affect this microbiome in our gut. The most significant effect is the reduction of the cyclical fluctuations that occur daily. This, in turn, can help reset the composition of our microbiome and restore key microbiota to improve all aspects of our health, including our cardiovascular health.

I also came upon a review with the purpose of providing an overview of all the most recent intermittent fasting literature, especially in terms of how it can affect cardiometabolic health (Antoni, et. al., 2014). Here are some highlights of this review:

- In individuals who had a healthy weight, following intermittent fasting for two to three weeks might not have a significant effect on their blood pressure or resting heart rate.
- In terms of gender-specific effects of intermittent fasting over the course of three weeks, changes in the levels of HDL cholesterol were only observed in females. On the other hand, decreases in triglyceride levels were only observed in males.

While many studies have shown promising results, there are a few which suggest inconsistencies such as these. As such, the best course of action is for the experts to continue doing further research on the benefit of IF on cardiovascular health to ease the minds of those who are interested in following the eating pattern to specifically improve their cardiovascular health.

REDUCES THE RISK OF CANCER

By now, you may have noticed that intermittent fasting has a protective effect on the body. This is a very important benefit as it can prevent the development of various diseases, even cancer. Among all diseases, cancer is one of the worst. This terrible disease is mainly characterized by the uncontrolled growth of cancerous cells. If you cannot control this growth through treatment or other kinds of interventions, the disease will just keep getting worse.

Fortunately, intermittent fasting offers a number of metabolic benefits that can help reduce the risk of cancer. There aren't many studies conducted on humans that focus on this benefit. However, there are several animal studies that show promising results in terms of the prevention of this debilitating disease. In one particular study, the researchers found out that fasting may help protect the healthy cells in the bodies of mice from the adverse side effects of the drugs administered during chemotherapy (Lee, et. al., 2012). This effect can potentially apply to humans too. According to the study, multiple fasting cycles can promote the differential sensitization of stress in tumors. This intervention even has the potential to augment or replace the efficacy of specific drugs administered during chemotherapy.

Although the scientific side of this benefit is still in its infancy, the power of intermittent fasting in the prevention or reduction of the risk of cancer lies in its effects on the cells. The general underlying theory of IF in terms of cancer is how it helps our cells adapt to stress. It is believed that healthy cells are more efficient at adapting to a lack of nutrients compared to cancer cells. The latter needs to consume a lot of nutrients to grow. Of course, if you alternate between cycles of eating and fasting, this means that while fasting, you will be starving the cancer cells too. Furthermore, if you are undergoing chemotherapy treatment while following IF, this could increase the susceptibility of the cancer cells to DNA damage and oxidative stress. In other words, IF can potentially make the cancer cells more sensitive to chemotherapy treatment.

More evidence is pointing to the effectiveness of fasting for a period of 18 hours and allowing yourself to eat normally for the remaining 6 hours. According to experts, this might be the ideal ratio for your body to trigger the "metabolic switch" where your body starts burning fat instead of glucose. When your body is in this state, you experience a greater resistance to stress, improved longevity, and a decreased risk of developing various diseases, including cancer. One particular study showed that when obese mice were placed on IF, this reduced the accumulation of fat in their livers, decreased the inflammatory expression of their genes, and reduced their risk of cancer (Varady & Hellerstein, 2007). For this benefit, there have been numerous studies conducted on animals, and here are some highlights of the most interesting ones that I have read:

- One study has indicated that intermittent fasting can help decrease the spontaneous occurrence of tumors in rats (de Cabo & Mattson, 2019).
- Another study has reported that intermittent fasting can help prevent cancer cells from metabolizing energy, thus, hindering their growth and making them more vulnerable to treatments such as chemotherapy (O'Flanagan, et. al., 2017). This same study also suggested that intermittent fasting can help decrease the side effects that may come from certain cytotoxic treatments.

While most studies focused on animals, there was one that focused on the effect of intermittent fasting on people who suffered from breast and ovarian cancer who were undergoing chemotherapy (Bauersfeld, et. al., 2018). This study raised my spirits as it was done on humans, not rats. Here, the participants had to start their fast 36 hours before their chemotherapy session then end it 24 hours after their chemotherapy session. After the trial, the participants who underwent fasting experienced less fatigue, along with an improvement in their quality of life during their chemotherapy sessions. All of these studies are indeed promising, and hopefully, there will be more to provide concrete and consistent evidence on how IF can prevent or improve different types of cancer.

SUPPORTS NEUROLOGICAL HEALTH

Whether this benefit has crossed your mind or not, it is one of the most important benefits of intermittent fasting. If we want to live long, happy, and productive lives, we should also focus on maintaining our neurological health. Intermittent fasting proves to be one of the best diet choices you can make as it can also support the health of the nervous system, enhances cognitive function, and helps reduce the risk of developing neurodegenerative diseases. These benefits come from the restricted eating times that come with intermittent fasting.

Generally, anything that improves the health of your body would also improve the health of your brain. The metabolic benefits of intermittent fasting, such as the reduction of inflammation, oxidative stress, and blood sugar levels, are all important for neurological health. As with all the other benefits, there have been several animal studies conducted that show how intermittent fasting can be beneficial for the brain. For instance, one study has shown that intermittent fasting can help with the process known as neurogenesis—the process by which the neural stem cells produce neurons (Lee, et. al., 2000). This study and similar ones provide valuable insight in terms of how diet can affect the plasticity of the brain to prevent the development of neurodegenerative disorders.

In another study, the researchers discovered that intermittent fasting may promote the production of a brain hormone known as brain-derived neurotrophic factor or BDNF (Mattson, 2005). This is significant since a deficiency of BDNF is associated with different brain issues like depression. An increase in the levels of BDNF in the brain also strengthens neuronal resistance to avoid degeneration and dysfunction. There was also a study related to this brain hormone, but this time, it focused on Huntington's disease (Duan, et. al., 2003). People who suffer from this disease have low levels of BDNF. Since intermittent fasting can help increase the production of this hormone, it can be an excellent dietary intervention for carriers of the mutant huntingtin gene. It can potentially prevent the disease from developing, thus, increasing the lifespan of those who carry the gene.

Intermittent fasting doesn't just protect the brain—it can also improve brain structures and cognitive functions. These were the results of one study done on mice (Liaoliao, et. al., 2013). In a separate animal study, the researchers discovered that intermittent fasting could potentially protect the brain against Alzheimer's disease (Zhang, et. al., 2017). People who suffer from Alzheimer's disease have an excessive accumulation of the protein amyloid-β (Aβ) in their brains. If this accumulation can be avoided or cleared up, it can help prevent or improve the disease. The results of the study showed that intermittent fasting could help prevent the accumulation of Aβ in the brain, thus, preventing the risk of developing the disease. Since intermittent fasting is relatively easy to follow, this can be suggested for the prevention of Alzheimer's disease.

Although fasting has been around for a long time now, scientists and researchers have yet to explore all the potential benefits and applications, especially in terms of the debilitating neurological diseases that plague our world today. But what we do know is that intermittent fasting induces a different kind of metabolic state that improves the resilience, bioenergetics, and plasticity of the neurons in our brains. This fact and all the promising results of the studies that focus on the brain health benefit of intermittent fasting show us that this eating pattern is good for our most important organ. Over time, you may experience improvement in your cognitive skills. Intermittent fasting may even improve the functional recovery of the brain for people who have experienced a brain injury or stroke. Hopefully, we will continue hearing about studies that solidify the claims and make us feel more confident in this benefit of intermittent fasting.

AUTOPHAGY

Autophagy is an essential mechanism in the body wherein the old, damaged, and dead organic materials (like proteins, cell membranes, organelles, and so on) are recycled to repair or create healthy cells. In other words, this is a natural, regulated process that degrades and recycles cellular components. Autophagy is the body's way of clearing out useless materials to create newer and healthier cells. You want this process to happen within your body because it comes with its own host of health benefits. One of the most effective ways to trigger autophagy is through intermittent fasting.

The key activator of this bodily mechanism is nutrient deprivation. Remember that fasting causes your insulin levels to go down, especially when your body has already used up all the glucose from the last meal you consumed. When your body's insulin levels go down, the production of a hormone called glucagon increases. This increase activates the process of autophagy. As this process is activated, you also experience an increase in your growth hormone levels. This means that as autophagy clears out all unnecessary cellular components, your body also works hard to produce new cells. It's like your body is undergoing a much-needed renovation.

One study has shown how nutrient restriction is key to the activation of autophagy (Antunes, et. al., 2018). Since nutrient restriction occurs regularly when you follow intermittent fasting, this means that your body will undergo autophagy regularly too. Here are some benefits this process offers:

- It helps with the regulation of the mitochondria of cells to improve the production of energy.
- It encourages the growth of nerve and brain cells while providing a protective effect on the entire nervous system.

- It encourages the growth of heart cells while protecting you against heart disease.
- It provides a protective effect on DNA stability.
- It gives your immune system a boost by getting rid of intracellular pathogens.
- It prevents healthy organs and tissues from getting damaged.
- It has the potential to combat neurodegenerative diseases, cancer, and other types of illnesses.

Fasting increases the rate of apoptosis (cell death) along with autophagy. This is another natural process that helps to improve our health. After the cells die, autophagy starts recycling the components of those cells. Then comes the renewal of cells and even the production of new cells. Of course, the longer your fasting period is, the longer these processes can continue working. However, as soon as you eat something, these processes all come to a halt.

There was one study done that revealed an important aspect of this process (Mihaylova, et. al., 2018). Here, the researchers discovered the oxidation of fatty acids inside the cells' mitochondria actually improves the function of our stem cells. This is a very important benefit since our stem cells tend to lose their efficiency as we age. Since autophagy can help renew these cells and intermittent fasting activates this metabolic process, this means that autophagy also has a positive impact on aging and our overall health.

Of course, this is just one study. But one thing is for sure—autophagy is an essential process in the body to keep you young, renewed, and healthy. There is a lot more to this process for you to learn about, and you can do this by going online and doing research about it. I have shared with you the basics of autophagy and how it can benefit the body in relation to intermittent fasting. But being a complex process in itself, you can understand it better by learning more about it. What I can say for now is that intermittent fasting is an important stimulator of autophagy. This, in turn, also allows you to enjoy all of the benefits autophagy has to offer.

OTHER HEALTH BENEFITS

I could go on and on about the benefits of intermittent fasting. But I have already shared the most significant ones, and with this last point, I will go through a few others. Intermittent fasting is wonderful as it stimulates a number of changes in the body to optimize the way it works. Here are some other benefits that could be linked to intermittent fasting according to various studies:

Reduces Inflammation

This benefit of intermittent fasting can help in the prevention or management of pro-inflammatory conditions. Although IF provides this benefit, it doesn't have a negative effect on the response of the immune system to acute infections. Caloric restriction has pro-inflammatory effects, as shown in one study (Jordan, et. al., 2019). Although the results of this study have shown that intermittent fasting can reduce inflammation, the mechanisms by which this occurs aren't completely understood yet. What the researchers know for sure is that the reduction of inflammation can help improve chronic inflammatory diseases. The results of this study were supported by an older study that also showed how intermittent fasting could combat inflammation (Johnson, et. al., 2007). In this older study, the researchers focused on how this benefit can improve our quality of life since inflammation is one of the major causes of different types of diseases and disorders.

Reduces Oxidative Damage

This benefit comes from the process of autophagy. When intermittent fasting stimulates autophagy, the process then repairs your cells to improve cell survival. There are many factors that cause oxidative damage, but when your cells are strengthened, this increases their ability to resist oxidative stress and damage more effectively. Just like inflammation, oxidative stress is one of the risk factors of several chronic diseases. Fortunately, several studies have shown how intermittent fasting may increase your body's oxidative stress resistance (Mattson & Wan, 2004). In another study that focused on aging mechanisms, the researchers suggested that caloric restriction can prolong one's lifespan (Weindruch & Sohal, 2010). This also happens when our cells and our whole body becomes stronger and more resistant to oxidative damage. When you restrict calories through intermittent fasting, different processes kick in, all of which work together to improve your health.

Potentially Improves Aerobic Capacity

Finally, intermittent fasting can also be beneficial to athletes and to those who lead an active lifestyle. For instance, when you choose the alternate-day fasting method, this can increase your endurance and your aerobic capacity since your body will switch to fat-burning instead of glucose-burning. This benefit on endurance is what the researchers observed in mice after they put the mice on the diet for a specific period of time (Marosi, et. al., 2018). The results of this study suggest that fasting intermittently can help rats (and potentially, even humans) reach optimum performance while maintaining good health. The researchers also encouraged further study to prove this fact.

Another study conducted on mice also showed how intermittent fasting helped improve their aerobic capacity (Chaix, et. al., 2014). Here, the mice that followed IF were able to run 60 minutes longer than mice that had access to food all day even though they approximately weighed the same. Then there is the weight loss benefit of intermittent fasting to consider along with the fact that this eating pattern doesn't promote muscle loss. All of these factors contribute to the potential improvement of aerobic capacity.

As you can see, intermittent fasting offers so many significant benefits to your health. Even if you just wanted to shed some excess pounds, you will also see an improvement in your overall health as you continue to stick with this eating pattern. One important thing that you can take away from this chapter is that IF has a lot of potential benefits. Even though most of the studies I have presented were conducted on animals, they have shown incredibly promising results. In the near future, we might hear about human studies that show similar or even better results. As you follow IF, keep an eye on updates in terms of the benefits so that you can use these as one of your motivations to keep going.

3

THE MOST POPULAR WAYS TO DO INTERMITTENT FASTING

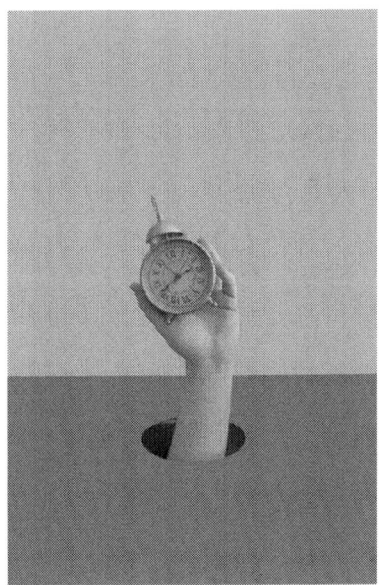

Fig. 4: IF Methods. Unsplash, by Elena Koycheva, 2018, https://unsplash.com/photos/VmcIMhuWCac/ Copyright 2018 by Elena Koycheva/Unsplash.

These days, fasting isn't just done for religious purposes or as part of a tradition. Today, people fast so that they can lose weight, improve their health or even as part of their treatment. Intermittent fasting has become a huge trend in recent years. All around the world, people have been following this eating pattern and because of its effectiveness, the same people have also been singing its praises. Intermittent fasting isn't a diet. It is more of an eating pattern where you would cycle between periods of fasting and eating.

The length and time that these periods happen would depend on the IF method you have chosen. There are several methods of intermittent fasting to choose from but the ones we will discuss here are the most common and popular ones. If it is your first time fasting intermittently, you can start with one of the easier methods and build up gradually to the more intense ones as your body adjusts to intermittent fasting. You can also give the different methods a try to see which one you can follow long-term.

One of the things that I love about intermittent fasting is its flexibility. Even if you have chosen a certain method, you can still customize it to fit into your schedule. This is also one reason why I found it quite easy to adjust to intermittent fasting. The first time I followed it, I made sure that my fasting window included my sleeping time. That way, I had seven to eight hours each day where I didn't have to feel hungry or think about how many hours were left until my next feeding window.

Of course, there were still times when I felt like I wanted to give in to my hunger and once in a while, I did. I indulged in a light snack whenever I felt like I couldn't focus on anything else or when I felt too lightheaded to function. Although allowing myself to give in to my hunger once in a while made me feel bad, I still tried to forgive myself to make things easier. If you're like me and it's your first time fasting, then you might experience challenges similar to this. But if you have had experience with fasting, then your journey might be smoother and easier.

For you to start your intermittent fasting journey, you must first decide which method to follow. To do this, it's recommended that you learn everything you can about the different methods. That way, you can try to determine which one might fit into your lifestyle best and give it a try. Try to pick at least two or three options so that you can shift to a new method if you think that the first one you have chosen isn't working for you. Now, let's go through the different methods to give you a better idea of what your options are.

5:2 METHOD

This is the most common intermittent fasting method. This IF method is also known as the Fast Diet and it was made popular by Michael Mosley, the British journalist. In a nutshell, this method involves fasting twice a week then eating normally for the rest of the days. This is a very flexible method because you can choose which days you will fast and which days you will eat normally. The only rule you would have to follow when you choose this method is that there should be at least one non-fasting day between your fasting days. In other words, this means that you shouldn't fast for two days straight.

During your fasting days, you would only consume a maximum of 500 calories. Although counting calories isn't a requirement on IF, this practice may help increase your chances of success, especially during your fasting windows. Over time, you will get a good sense of what a 500-calorie meal looks or feels like once you eat it. But in the beginning, counting calories can be very helpful. So if you should only be eating 500 calories on your fasting days, here are some examples of ways to plan to eat your meals:

- You can have a 200-calorie beef cheeseburger with the works (and the bun) in the morning and a 300-calorie hearty winter soup in the afternoon.
- You can start your day with a 300-calorie stir-fry rice bowl with shrimp or chicken then have a lighter 200-calorie meal of fajitas later in the afternoon.
- You can also stick with your 3-meals-a-day plan where you would eat 200-calorie turkey tacos for breakfast, 200-calorie baked tilapia with vegetables for lunch, and a 100-calorie salad for dinner.

As long as you stick with the 500 calories on your fasting days, choosing when to consume your meals is entirely up to you.

However, if you're following this method, it might not be the best option to eat a single 500-calorie meal for your fasting days, especially when you're still starting out. On the days when you aren't fasting, you should eat normally. If you can reduce the number of times you eat—like if you avoid snacking if you don't feel hungry—this might make your fasting days a lot easier. Just make sure that you don't eat more than what you normally do while convincing yourself that it's okay because, on your fasting days, you will be reducing your caloric intake.

Many people believe that this is the easiest IF method to follow. After all, you would only have to fast for 2 days each week and on those days, you won't have to fast completely. You can eat up to 500 calories on those days and you can choose how to spread out your meals. Of course, this method would be much more effective if you choose healthy meals, especially during your fasting days.

The 5:2 method might seem simple and easy, but when you're starting out, you will definitely feel the difference. This is especially true if you are used to eating more than the recommended number of calories each day. This is why you should plan your meals well throughout the day. This is also why it's important to drink regularly to keep yourself hydrated so you won't feel the intensity of your hunger pangs. Also, if you work out, play sports or have high-intensity training sessions, make sure that these strenuous activities don't fall on your fasting days. Otherwise, you might fall ill or even experience the other potential side effects of intermittent fasting. Choose your fasting days wisely to make it easier for you to follow this method.

16:8 METHOD

For this method, you would be fasting daily. Your feasting window would range between 14 to 16 hours giving you a feeding window between eight to ten hours. As with the 5:2 method, you decide when to schedule your fasting windows and feeding windows. Also, you can decide how many meals you want to eat within your feeding window. You can have two large meals, three smaller meals or even four light meals throughout your feeding window. One of the easiest ways to start on this method is by skipping your first or last meal of the day. Let me share an example of how you would create a schedule for following this IF method:

- You can skip breakfast so that your feeding window starts at 10:00 in the morning.
- Let's say that you plan to eat three meals throughout the day. This means that your first meal would be at 10:00 am.
- Your second meal could be around 1:00 or 2:00 in the afternoon.
- Your final meal would be at around 5:00 or 5:30 in the afternoon.
- At 6:00 in the evening, your fasting window begins

and it will end at 10:00 in the morning of the next day.

It looks simple, doesn't it? The 16:8 method is another easy IF method to follow and it's recommended for beginners. If you don't think that you can fast for 16 hours a day, then you can opt for the 14:10 method—a variation of this method. The 14:10 method may be more realistic and easier for you to follow because you would have an extra two hours for your feeding window. Using the same example as above, your day might look like this:

- You can skip breakfast so that your feeding window starts at 9:00 in the morning.
- Since your feeding time has been extended, you can plan to eat four meals throughout the day. This means that your first meal would be at 9:00 am.
- Your second meal could be around 12:00 noon.
- Then you can have a light snack around 3:00 in the afternoon.
- Your final meal would be at around 6:00 or 6:30 in the afternoon.
- At 7:00 in the evening, your fasting window begins and it will end at 9:00 in the morning of the next day.

Of course, if you're an early bird, you can start your feeding window at an earlier time. The key here is to eat what you want and need to within your feeding window, whether you choose eight or ten hours. If you have a day job, you can choose to set your feeding window at the same time as your working hours. That way, you will have the energy to work productively throughout the day. And when you go home, all you have to do is relax, wind down, and go to sleep.

Since this method involves fasting every day, it may take some time for you to find the perfect schedule. For instance, if you decide to set your feeding window at the same time as your working hours, you might discover that you're too busy to have time to eat. When this happens, your fasting window might end up being too long. In such a case, then you might have to move your feeding window to a different schedule—one where you can guarantee that you can eat enough to stay healthy each day. This method is relatively simple and it's not as extreme as the others. Therefore, you can try it out even if you have no prior fasting experience.

ALTERNATE-DAY FASTING METHOD

This method is like a different version of the 5:2 method. Instead of setting fasting and feeding windows for yourself, you would fast on alternate days. This means that every other day, you would eat regularly. Then on the days in between, you would have a fasting day wherein you restrict your caloric intake. To follow this method, you won't fast completely on your fasting days. Instead, you will reduce your caloric intake significantly—by around 70% to 75%. For instance, if your normal caloric intake for the day is 1,800 calories (on your normal eating days), then you would reduce this to 450 calories on your fasting days. Let me share an example of how your week would go as you start following this method:

- On Monday, you consume your normal 1,800 calories throughout the day.
- On Tuesday, you aim for only 450 calories. You can have a heavy 300-calorie meal in the morning and a lighter 150-calorie meal in the afternoon or early in the evening.
- On Wednesday, you go back to consuming your normal 1,800 calories throughout the day.
- On Thursday, you go back to 450 calories. You can have a light breakfast, lunch, and dinner wherein each meal only contains 150 calories.
- On Friday, you consume 1,800 calories spread throughout your day.
- On Saturday, you limit yourself to 450 calories again. This time, you can have a light 200-calorie meal in the morning and the evening with an even lighter 50-calorie snack in between.
- On Sunday, you go back to your normal 1,800 calories.

For the next week, you would switch the schedule as Monday becomes a fasting day. You can continue alternating between normal and fasting days if it works for you. You may have noticed that I provided different options for your fasting days. You can do this too. Find out what works best for you by trying out different things. If you think that consuming two meals on your fasting days is enough, stick with it. If not, then you can try a different approach.

For some people, this method is too difficult to follow. Usually, they are referring to the more advanced version of this method wherein fasting days are days when you literally fast, thus consuming zero calories. Throughout the day, you only drink water and other non-caloric drinks. As a beginner, I don't recommend this for you. Even if you have experience with fasting in the past, doing it every other day one week after another isn't recommended. Remember that fasting changes the way your body works. Although these changes can lead to a lot of health benefits, shocking your body by trying to fast for long periods of time and too frequently, you might end up compromising your health.

If you want to move forward with IF, it's best to start off slow. For instance, you can start with this method by just restricting your caloric intake on fasting days. When your body has adjusted to the caloric restriction, then you can reduce your food intake on your normal days by just a bit. For instance, if you normally consume 1,800 calories, you can bring this down to 1,600 calories. Follow this eating pattern for about a month or so to give your body time to adjust. Then you can try reducing your caloric intake on your fasting days. For instance, instead of consuming 450 calories, you can bring this down to 350 or 400 calories.

You need to go through a process of adjustment if you want to get the best results and if you want this eating pattern to work for you. These small modifications help your body adjust to intermittent fasting more effectively, thus, making the eating pattern more sustainable for you. You also have the choice to start with a different method and shift to the more advanced version of this one. The flexibility of IF means that you can try different methods until you find the method (and the variation) that suits your own lifestyle.

EAT-STOP-EAT METHOD

This method is one of the more intense ones, thus making it more challenging. Although I don't recommend it for you if you're an IF beginner, it's still worth learning about in case you will shift into this method in the future. This method is also known as the 24-hour fast because it involves fasting for one whole day. Typically, you would perform these 24-hour fasts once or twice each week. So the name of this method is quite literal as you will eat for a few days, stop for a day, eat again, and stop... eat-stop-eat.

This method is considered more difficult because it involves a full 24-hour period of not consuming anything at all. To keep your hunger at bay, you can only consume plain coffee, plain tea, water, and any other zero-calorie beverages you can find. As with the 5:2 method, you should have a non-fasting day between your 24-hour fasts. Going for two whole days without eating anything could lead to a number of adverse effects, therefore, this isn't recommended. For this method, let me give you an example of how your typical week would go:

- On Monday, you eat normally and dinner would be your last meal.
- On Tuesday, you have breakfast at 8:00 in the morning and nothing else. This is when your fast starts. For the rest of the day, you won't eat anything.
- On Wednesday, you end your fast by having breakfast at 9:00 in the morning to complete the 24-hour fast. Then you eat normally for the rest of the day.
- On Thursday, you again eat normally throughout the day.
- On Friday, you still continue eating normally throughout the day.
- On Saturday, you have breakfast at 8:00 in the morning then start your second 24-hour fast of the week. This means that you won't eat anything for the rest of the day.
- On Sunday, you have breakfast around 9:00 to end

your fast. Then you continue eating normally for the rest of the day.

This is just an example of how you can schedule your fasting days. Here, the fasting days are on Tuesday and Saturday. You can also choose the time when you start your fasting day. For instance, your last meal can be at lunchtime on your fasting day and this would continue until lunchtime the next day. Plan your schedule accordingly so that it becomes easier for you to follow. As with the other methods, it's best to set your fasting days when you know that your schedule won't be too busy and you won't have to perform any strenuous activities.

Since this method is similar to the 5:2 method, it can be the next step you take after following 5:2 for a couple of weeks or months. If you follow the 5:2 method, your body would eventually get used to eating fewer calories for two days each week. Then you can start reducing the number of calories on these days until you can eliminate all calories completely. This is just a suggestion for how you can advance from one method to another. At the end of the day, the decision still lies with you. For instance, if you try following this method for a few weeks and you notice some negative side effects (we'll discuss these later), then you might want to try a method that isn't as extreme.

Of course, if you think that you are ready for 24-hour fasts, you can try them out. If this method makes you feel better or you think that it's helping you reach your health and fitness goals, good for you! Just make sure that your body can sustain this eating pattern without increasing your risk of developing nutrient deficiencies, headaches, and other health issues.

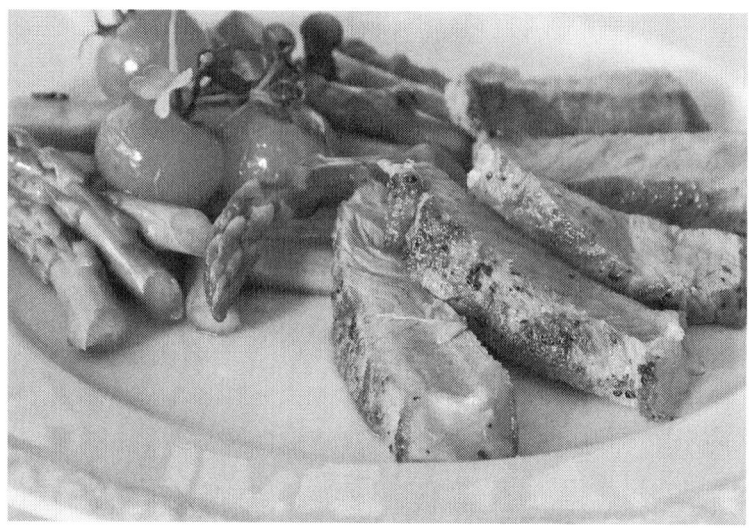

Fig. 5: OMAD. Pixabay, by RitaE, 2017, https://pixabay.com/ photos/asparagus-steak-veal-steak-veal-2169305/ Copyright 2017 by RitaE/Pixabay.

ONE MEAL A DAY METHOD

This method is the one that I am following now, and it also happens to be the main focus of this book. The name is pretty self-explanatory as this method involves eating only one meal each day. It's the perfect method for those who lead busy lifestyles or for those who want to give the more extreme methods of intermittent fasting a try. One thing I can tell you right now is that this isn't a method for beginners. Since you will be only eating a single meal each day, you have to plan your meal well.

For a lot of people, they can only eat so much in a single sitting. But if you only eat a "regular meal" like two pieces of chicken, a serving of mashed potatoes, and a glass of juice for the day, you'll definitely feel intense hunger pangs. Also, eating only one small meal every day could lead to nutrient deficiencies, so you should approach this method with enough practical knowledge and a lot of caution.

This method is sometimes called the 23:1 method as it involves 23 hours of fasting and only 1 hour of eating. But the truth is, you can take as long as you want to eat your meal as long as you eat it in a single sitting. If you're in a rush, you might even finish your meal in less than an hour. After your one meal of the day, you can only consume zero-calorie beverages for the rest of the day. If you're like me, you can start following this diet by counting calories. I did this because I wanted to make sure that I wasn't depriving myself. But again, this isn't a requirement. Many people believe that this is the simplest method to follow because all you have to do is eat a single meal each day. As long as the meal you have eaten makes you feel full and satisfied, then it has served its purpose.

Among all the methods of intermittent fasting, this is the one that involves the most caloric restriction in terms of quantity and consistency. No matter how hungry you are, you can only eat so much in a single sitting. So it's quite a challenge to overeat when following this method. Because of this caloric restriction, this method can result in sustainable weight loss along with all of the other benefits linked to intermittent fasting. Personally, I did lose a lot of weight when I started on OMAD. Although I already lost a significant amount of weight when I began my intermittent fasting diet, I did shed even more weight through this method.

One of the first tips I will share with you about OMAD is to focus on healthy foods. Since you will only be eating one meal, make sure it counts. Imagine what would happen to your body if your single meal of the day would always be something greasy, processed or high in sugar. Eating food like this every day and nothing else won't lead to health improvements, but the opposite. If you have already been following IF for some time now and you're ready to switch to OMAD, I will be sharing tips and strategies to help you succeed. The same thing goes for if you're planning to shift to OMAD after allowing your body to adjust to intermittent fasting through one of the easier methods first. When you're ready to start the OMAD routine, then you can apply everything that you will learn in the remaining chapters of this book. But before that, let me share with you the last method that you can start off with.

SPONTANEOUS MEAL SKIPPING METHOD

This final method I will share with you isn't technically considered a method of IF. But for someone who has never tried fasting before, this is the easiest and most relaxed way to start experiencing intermittent fasting. For this method, you would spontaneously skip meals whenever you feel like it. For instance, if you're too busy at work, you decide to skip lunch. Or dinnertime comes, and you're not hungry, you decide to skip dinner and do something else instead. Each time you skip one of your regular meals, this allows you to engage in a certain fasting period. Let me share a more specific example for you:

- In the morning, you start your day with a healthy breakfast.
- Come lunchtime, you have a lot of things to do at work, so you decide to grab a light salad for a quick lunch.
- At around 4:00 in the afternoon, you feel hungry, so you eat a burrito as a snack.
- When it's time for dinner, you still feel full from the burrito you ate, so you decide to have a glass of water before starting your bedtime routine.
- You go to bed and the next morning, you have breakfast at 7:00.

This is a perfect example of spontaneous meal skipping. In this example, the last meal you had was your snack at 4:00 in the afternoon. This means that you would have fasted from around 5:00 in the afternoon to 7:00 in the morning the next day. Although it may have been a spontaneous decision to skip your last meal of the day, you would have already given yourself a fasting window of 14 hours!

For beginners, this is an excellent method because you don't have to follow a strict or structured nutritional regimen. It will just be like giving yourself a chance to practice fasting intermittently without making any commitments yet. Then when you feel like you have gotten the hang of fasting, you can choose one of the IF methods that have flexible rules.

This is also a great option if you eat instinctively. If you're used to eating only when you feel hungry, this method allows you to skip meals whenever you don't feel hungry. If you had already been doing this in the past, that means that you were already following IF on some level. Now, it might be the right time for you to give the other methods a try. Meal skipping is a great way to start your IF journey, but at some point, you should try to make your fasting windows more of a regular thing. That way, you will really train your body to learn how to survive without eating anything for certain periods of time.

As you can see, all of the IF methods are simple and easy to follow. They offer flexibility in terms of when you set the time or day of your fasting window. At this point, you should already have a good idea of which methods can potentially be the ones you choose for your IF journey. Since this book is all about the OMAD method, we will be going into more detail about it in the next chapter. Whether you have chosen this method to follow or you want to try the other methods too, the tips you will learn in the next chapters will also be very helpful for you. So, keep turning those pages!

4

ONE MEAL A DAY METHOD OF INTERMITTENT FASTING

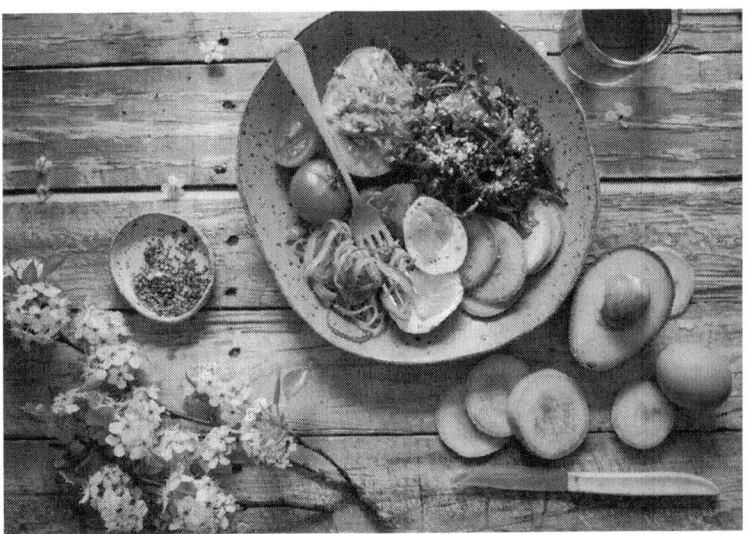

Fig. 6: All About OMAD. Unsplash, by Brooke Larke, 2017, https://unsplash.com/photos/jUPOXXRNdcA/ Copyright 2017 by Brooke Larke/Unsplash.

The One Meal A Day method of intermittent fasting is considered as one of the most extreme methods. But it also happens to be one of the most popular IF methods, especially for those who want to get stellar results in a short amount of time. As I have mentioned in the last chapter, this method is more challenging than the others, especially if you're an IF beginner or if you have never tried fasting before. Still, having been a follower of this diet for quite some time now, I can tell you that there are things you can do to make your OMAD intermittent fasting journey a lot easier.

If your main goal is to lose a lot of weight, OMAD is one of the best methods for you. Of course, this isn't the only benefit you will get from following OMAD. You can look forward to all the other benefits of IF through this method too. But following it entails some education and planning, especially if it's your first time and you want to succeed. As the name implies, you will only eat a single meal each day on OMAD. The flexibility of intermittent fasting comes in the form of the time when you eat your single meal. For instance, if you eat a big, satisfying breakfast, then you won't consume anything until the next day.

It's important to note that "one meal" in this method doesn't mean that you should eat a regular meal. For instance, if your normal meal consists of a scoop of mashed potatoes, a piece of roasted chicken, and a side of buttered veggies, this can tide you over until your next meal. However, if you're on OMAD, you may want to increase your caloric intake a bit. Remember—the single meal you eat should be enough to make you feel full and satisfied. Although it's not recommended to strive to overeat for your one meal of the day, it's also not recommended to pair this method with severe caloric restriction. Fasting is different from starving and you shouldn't aim for the latter.

As a proponent of the OMAD method, I can tell you how it has made my life a lot simpler and easier. I only have to worry about eating one meal a day, but I always make sure that it makes me feel full, satisfied, and happy. I take my one meal at dinner so that I have time to prepare the ingredients for it, cook the dish, and enjoy eating it. After my meal, I relax, wind down, and get ready for bed. No matter how busy I am in the day, no matter how stressful my day has been, this single meal (and the routine that goes with it) makes my days complete. Although I tried following other methods in the past, when I started on OMAD, I realized that I had found the method that was perfect for my own lifestyle. From this chapter, you will learn everything that there is to know about OMAD, and you will have a better idea if this could be the perfect method for you too.

WHY IS OMAD CONSIDERED THE BEST METHOD OF INTERMITTENT FASTING?

When those who know all about IF hear that you follow the OMAD method, they'll think you're hardcore. This is because most people won't purposely choose to only eat one meal for the whole day, every day. However, there is historic evidence that suggests that this method of eating has been around for centuries. Some records even suggest that the Romans only consumed one meal each day. For them, digestion was such an important bodily process that they considered eating more than once each day to be a form of gluttony. For a long time, this belief had an influence on their eating patterns.

In other parts of Europe back in the middle ages, breakfast wasn't considered part of their day. Although most people believe that this is the most important part of the day, even the monarchs in Europe rarely ate this morning meal. Instead, the people in those times had their first meal of the day late in the morning—around 10:00 am or 11:00 am—then have their second meal a few hours later. In the past, people didn't eat as frequently as most people eat now. Back then, this type of eating was a normal part of their lives.

Now, OMAD is making a comeback as more and more people are getting interested in following this extreme yet effective eating pattern. Of course, OMAD isn't a perfect diet nor is it a diet that's suitable for everyone. Because of the nature of this method, you must first think carefully about your current health and eating patterns so that you can determine whether it would be right for you. But, despite all of the potential risks, it still remains to be one of the emerging methods of IF that is gaining more followers. We have already discussed the general benefits of intermittent fasting in Chapter 2. Now, let's take a look at some reasons why the OMAD method is considered to be the best:

Simplicity and convenience

This is the main benefit of OMAD and the reason why I love this eating pattern too. Once you get used to this method, you will discover that it involves minimal planning and preparation. Think about it: how much time do you need for meal planning when you eat three times a day? You have to think of fifteen different meals to prepare for the week for a five-day workweek. On OMAD, all you have to plan for is one meal each day. That reduces the meals you have to plan to only five each week, thus, cutting down your planning time significantly. This covers the convenient aspect of OMAD.

OMAD is also simple—just eat one meal a day. Then all you have to think about is what other things you can do for the day to make yourself as productive as possible. Just don't forget to hydrate yourself throughout the day to avoid any adverse side effects.

More intense health benefits

Since OMAD is an IF method, it means that it also offers the same general benefits as the other methods. But since this is a more advanced and intense method, you can also expect to experience more intense health benefits. Here are some examples:

- You may lose weight faster compared to other IF methods.
- Your human growth hormone levels increase, thus, allowing your body to burn fat while building muscle.
- Your inflammation levels may go down significantly along with your risk of developing certain diseases.
- You may experience an increase in autophagy, which, in turn, offers its own benefits.
- You may experience an improvement in your body's nutritional ketosis, which, in turn, comes with more fat-burning and anti-inflammatory benefits.

Basically, the OMAD method allows you to enjoy the benefits of intermittent fasting more intensely and at a faster rate. Since you will be fasting for longer periods of time each day, you can start feeling the benefits of IF sooner.

If you choose to follow the OMAD diet, try controlling your cravings. Resist your urge to scarf down anything and everything that you crave as soon as it's time for you to eat your one meal of the day. Instead, it's best to opt for healthy, whole foods as these will make you feel more full and more satisfied. Over time, you may notice that you aren't craving unhealthy foods as much as you did in the past. Eating healthily is a choice and the best time to make this choice is when you choose to follow the OMAD method.

THE BENEFITS OF THE OMAD METHOD

As simple as the OMAD method is, it can be quite challenging to follow, especially for first-timers. But with patience, commitment, and consistency, following this diet is entirely achievable. But if you're still on the fence about this extreme method, you may want to learn more about all the benefits it has to offer. OMAD gives you a chance to enjoy all of the benefits that IF has to offer simply because it is an IF method. But there are certain benefits that come with this method exclusively. Let's go through these now:

Fast and effective weight loss

Weight loss is the most sought-after benefit of intermittent fasting. Although this benefit can potentially come from all of the IF methods, you may experience it faster on OMAD. When you only eat a single meal each day, you will definitely be restricting your caloric intake. The great thing about the OMAD method is that it's quite challenging to overeat. For instance, if you have a feeding window of eight hours, you might feel tempted to eat frequently throughout that time. Convincing yourself that it's okay to eat a lot is much easier with a longer feeding window as you would tell yourself that your fasting window is longer anyway. But if you eat more calories than what you normally eat when you're not fasting, you might not see those excess pounds dropping off anytime soon.

On the other hand, when you're on OMAD, you have a maximum of one hour to eat your meal. For a single meal, this is already a lot of time. Usually, eating one satisfying meal will be enough for you, and when your hour is up, it's time for you to start fasting. Even if you use the whole hour to eat, there is a very small likelihood that you can consume all the calories you eat on a regular day at that time. If you do, you might end up feeling sick after!

Because of the very nature of the OMAD method, you will definitely be restricting your caloric intake—and you will do this every day. Naturally, this will cause you to lose weight. This fact was supported by the results of one study where the researchers discovered that the weight loss in people who fasted and people who restricted their overall caloric intake lost was almost the same (Templeman, et. al., 2019). Since OMAD involves fasting and caloric restriction, weight loss will come faster.

When it comes to weight loss sustainability, OMAD shines too. OMAD offers consistency in terms of the method by which you follow the diet. When you train yourself to eat just one meal a day, it becomes easier for your body to adjust. Since the other methods don't offer consistency, it might take more time for your body to adjust to the feeling of fasting. Even if you follow the other methods consistently (which is very important), OMAD is actually easier to adjust to because you will be doing the same thing every day. It's even better if you set your feeding window at the same time each day so you can make it part of your daily routine. When your body adjusts to the eating pattern, you feel more motivated to stick with it. This means that you will continue losing weight until you have reached your healthy weight and maintain it. This benefit was supported by a study wherein the researchers discovered that the participants were able to maintain their weight throughout the study's research period of 6 months (Stote, et. al., 2007). The study also showed that the participants who followed OMAD experienced a reduction in their fat mass. While losing weight is a general benefit of intermittent fasting, OMAD has the potential to improve this benefit compared to the other IF methods.

Better concentration and focus

Following OMAD can do wonders for your concentration and focus. This happens in two ways. First, because of the simplicity of this eating pattern, you don't have to think about where you will have your next meal, what you will eat, or how to budget your food allowance. After planning your one meal of the day, you have all the time to focus on other tasks.

You will feel these benefits, even more, when your body adjusts to the OMAD method. Your body achieves homeostasis once again. After the initial fatigue or weakness, you might experience at the beginning, and your energy levels will start going up. Then you will feel more focused no matter what you are doing, which, in turn, helps you concentrate better. And when it's time for you to have your meal of the day, you can focus on eating too. This makes the experience more satisfying.

Freedom from having to plan several meals throughout the day

This is the best benefit of OMAD for people who lead busy lives. Having to only plan a single meal each day is a relief. Even if you're used to meal planning, all you have to do is think about one meal each day. Shopping and cooking become easier too. And you don't have to resort to eating takeout frequently because you don't have time to prepare your meals. You can always ensure that what you are eating is healthy and nourishing.

You don't need to adhere to strict calorie restrictions

While it's not recommended to overeat while on OMAD, you don't have to restrict your caloric intake either. In fact, it's not recommended to restrict your caloric intake while following this method because you might end up developing nutrient deficiencies. Calorie restriction is the most difficult aspect of a diet. On OMAD, you won't feel like you are restricting yourself, especially if you make sure that your meal always makes you feel full and satisfied.

It might even help improve your performance

When you think of this method, you might not think that it would be suitable for those who live active lifestyles. But the fact is, there are some professional athletes who have started following OMAD to gain all the benefits. One such athlete is

Herschel Walker, the NFL star. He skips breakfast and lunch and only engages in long and intense training throughout the day. When dinner time comes, he eats his one meal of the day. Walker also happens to be a vegetarian, which means that his diet is plant-based. To Walker, it's all about the mindset. He has been eating this way for a long time now, and it makes life easier for him. In fact, he even believes that this type of lifestyle improves his performance. This is one example of how OMAD can also be suitable for you even if you work out or undergo training for sports competitions.

It helps improve your willpower and discipline

Finally, OMAD strengthens your willpower and discipline too. This eating method can be quite challenging, especially for beginners. Sticking with it for the long-run means that you should have a lot of discipline and self-control. Hunger pangs are very powerful, and if you give in to them all the time, you can't really follow this method. On the other hand, if you can master this extreme eating pattern, you will also be honing your willpower and discipline in the process.

As you can see, OMAD comes with a lot of great things too. It makes other IF methods look very easy, whether you are a beginner or not. As long as you learn how to follow it properly —don't worry, there aren't any strict rules, just a few guidelines and suggestions—you can experience all of these benefits and more.

HOW TO FOLLOW THE OMAD METHOD

The OMAD diet is relatively simple. Unlike diets, there aren't any strict rules that you must follow. But just like the other IF methods, OMAD comes with a few guidelines and suggestions that can help make your journey simpler and easier. For instance, it's best to choose a time for when you will have your meal of the day—try to stick with this time consistently. For instance, you can skip breakfast and dinner, and have a big meal at lunch. Personally, I skip breakfast and lunch, then have a big, satisfying dinner. This is the best time for me because I'm not busy, and I get to enjoy my meal without having to rush through it. Of course, the timing would be entirely up to you. Now, here are a few more tips to help you follow this extreme IF method:

1. Ease into the diet

Since this method is quite extreme, it's not recommended to jump right into it right away. For instance, after reading this book, you decide to start following OMAD tomorrow—without a plan and without prior experience. Instead, you may want to think of how you will approach this eating pattern first. Come up with a plan of your own for how to start following OMAD. Give yourself time to adjust to make things much easier for you.

2. Learn how to listen to your body

ONE MEAL A DAY METHOD OF INTERMITTENT FASTING | 75

Learning how to listen to your body is vital if you want to succeed on OMAD or on any other method of IF, for that matter. Even if you eat the healthiest meal each day, there are some bodies that don't do well with fasting for 23 hours each day. If you have such a body, then OMAD might not be the best choice for you. For instance, if you feel stressed all the time, your sleeping patterns are disturbed or you are constantly tired even after you have been following the method for a few months, then you may need to rethink your diet choices. You can modify your IF method based on how it makes your body feel, but you can only do this by learning how to listen to your body and all of its cues.

3. If you are a woman, be more careful

While everyone should practice caution when it comes to OMAD, women should be particularly careful. There have been cases where women experienced suppression of their reproductive hormones because of this extreme method. If you're a woman and you have noticed changes in your monthly cycle after following this eating pattern, have yourself checked. In fact, you may want to have yourself checked first before starting the OMAD method in the first place, especially if you also suffer from any medical condition.

4. Try to watch what you eat

Just because OMAD (and IF in general) focuses more on your timing and not the food that you eat, this doesn't mean that you should eat anything and everything that you want. For instance, having a single meal that consists of chips, fried chicken wings, and a mug of beer isn't the best type of meal to have on OMAD. Such a meal might make you feel full after eating it but it won't sustain you for the rest of the day.

Also, gorging on unhealthy foods every day will put you on a path that's far from the health and wellness goals you expect to achieve through intermittent fasting. As much as possible, it's best to opt for a nutrient-dense, balanced meal each day to ensure that your body is well-nourished. Once in a while, you may indulge in your food cravings. Just pair these with a healthy side dish like a salad to add nutrients to your meal.

5. Make sure your meal counts

Since you will only be having one meal for the day, make sure it counts. This is why I started OMAD by counting calories. Since I was trying to overcome a condition (insulin resistance), I had to make sure that I wasn't depriving myself of the nutrients my body needed to stay healthy. After some time, I didn't have to keep counting calories because I already had a good estimation of the caloric content of my meals. I learned how to prepare and cook my own meals too. This was very helpful. Instead of ordering out, I made sure that all my meals were balanced, healthy, nutrient-dense, satisfying, and they made me feel happy. Cooking my own meals also enabled me to gain a good estimation of the calories that different types of food contain.

6. Be flexible even with the timing

I suggested that you stick with a constant eating time to make it easier for your body to adjust to OMAD. However, this is only a suggestion. This way of eating has worked for me, but if it doesn't work for you, then find your own strategy. For instance, if you want to spread out your large meal over the course of an hour, do that. Or if you have decided to eat your meal at lunchtime but you already feel hungry at breakfast (maybe because you had a lot of activities on the previous day), allow yourself to eat. Don't let the schedule you have set; take control of your life. Being too strict with yourself might make you feel bad, which, in turn, might even push you to give up.

7. Try not to consume a lot of carbs

This is another suggestion that can improve your chances of succeeding in OMAD. Remember that one of the benefits of this eating pattern is autophagy. Also, fasting for long periods of time forces your body into ketosis for it to become an efficient fat-burning machine. However, when you eat a lot of carbs, your body won't achieve ketosis and autophagy until it has burned and used all of the starches and sugars from those carbs completely. Naturally, this will take a longer time if your meal is full of carbs like rice, pasta, bread, and other high-carb food sources. Instead, you may want to opt for healthy fats, proteins, and minimal carbs to make for a more satisfying and filling meal.

8. Know what to eat and what to avoid

In line with the last tip, it would also be a good idea for you to know what are the best foods to eat on OMAD and what are the foods you should limit or avoid. Even though intermittent fasting doesn't involve restricting yourself in terms of the foods you eat, choosing healthy foods will help you reach your health and fitness goals a lot faster. When planning your meals, here are some of the best options to include:

1. **Beverages** like fresh fruit juice, water, seltzer, etc.
2. **Broth**, preferably homemade.
3. **Condiments** like apple cider vinegar, olive oil, salt, pepper, etc.
4. **Dairy** like plain yogurt, cottage cheese, milk, etc.
5. **Fruits** like apples, bananas, mangoes, peaches, kiwis, etc.
6. **Herbs** like parsley, cilantro, basil, etc.
7. **Protein** like eggs, steak, turkey, chicken, fish, etc.
8. **Vegetables** like carrots, leafy greens, cauliflower, celery, garlic, mushrooms, broccoli, zucchini, etc.

You can also include small portions of the following when planning your meals:

1. **Grains** like quinoa, oats, pasta, etc.
2. **Nuts** like almonds, cashews, macadamias, etc.

3. **Seeds** like sunflower seeds, chia seeds, etc.
4. **Starches** like corn, potatoes, beans, etc.

Then there are the foods you may want to avoid, especially when planning your one meal for the day. These are the foods that you may allow yourself to indulge in occasionally, as long as you pair these foods with healthier options. The foods to avoid include:

1. Artificial sweeteners.
2. Cakes, cookies, and other sugary pastries.
3. Chips and other processed snacks.
4. Processed meats.
5. Refined carbs.
6. Sweetened or carbonated beverages with added sugar.
7. Sweets.

As long as you plan your meals well and you make sure that your meals contain all of the nutrients you need to stay healthy, you can eat whatever you want while on OMAD. Also, make sure that your meals make you feel happy and satisfied so that you won't be thinking about food for the rest of the day.

The OMAD method is so simple, but it helps to have a plan for following it. Also, the more you learn about OMAD, the more you can prepare yourself for what's about to come. So, for the last section of this chapter, let me give you a brief introduction of the "dark side" of OMAD to provide you with a clearer look at the whole picture.

THE POTENTIAL RISKS AND DOWNSIDES OF THE OMAD METHOD

We have already established that the OMAD diet is an eating pattern where you would eat one healthy, balanced, and satisfying meal per day within a span of one hour. But for some people, especially the ones who try following this method for the first time, they use their short feeding window to have a massive binge. Obviously, this is not the way to go. Binge eating is never good for your health and when you do it every day, you might experience a decline in your health instead of an improvement.

The OMAD method has a lot of potential benefits, and it's super-easy to follow. However, it's not perfect. As it is, you don't have to worry about the timing of your food because you will only eat one meal each day. This simplicity makes the diet seem too good to be true and for some people, it is. The potential risks and downsides of the OMAD method typically apply to those who don't follow this eating pattern correctly. Here are some examples of situations when OMAD can become troublesome instead of beneficial:

- Some people only eat unhealthy foods for their one meal. If you want the OMAD diet to work for you, it's

recommended to have a home-cooked meal that contains vitamins, minerals, and nutrients all in one plate (or bowl).
- Some people don't consume enough protein while focusing only on high-carb foods. This won't work because too many carbs will make you feel hungry after some time. Also, not consuming enough protein might put you at risk for muscle loss.
- Some people who suffer from a condition might need to take medications with their food. Of course, this will be a problem when they only eat one meal a day. In such a case, if you really want to follow OMAD, consult with your doctor first. Find out if there is any way for you to follow this method while still taking your medications.
- Some experts claim that OMAD can potentially slow down your metabolism in the long-run. This may happen if you follow OMAD for a long time as the slowing down of your metabolism is a natural response when you fast for long periods of time. This is why it's important to transition out of OMAD slowly—so that your body can adjust to the changes again.

To avoid the negative side effects of OMAD, your plate should contain the recommended daily amounts of vegetables, fruits, and protein in a single meal. Remember that this meal should be enough to tide you over until the next day. This is just a peek at the things that can go wrong with OMAD. Later, we will discuss these in more detail to help you understand them more. But before that, let me share with you the best tips and strategies for following OMAD (and IF) correctly. That way, you won't have to deal with the negative side effects and potential risks of this extreme method. When you know what to expect and how to overcome issues, there is a higher likelihood that you will succeed in your OMAD journey.

5

PREPARING TO FOLLOW THE OMAD METHOD OF INTERMITTENT FASTING

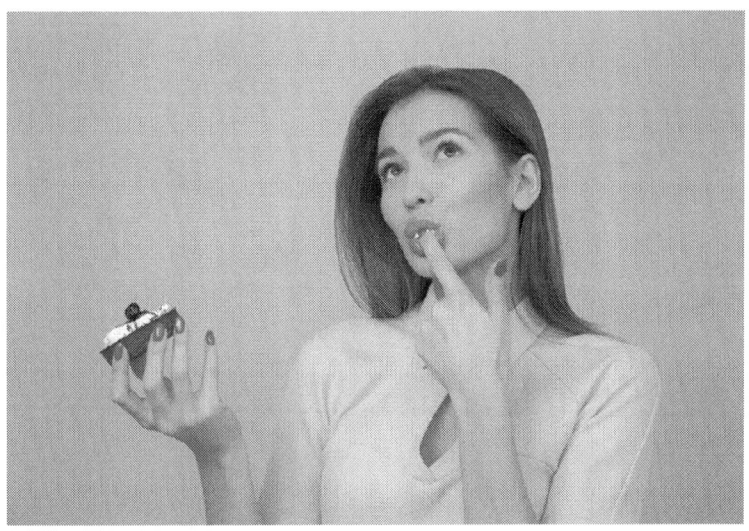

Fig. 7: Getting Ready for OMAD. Unsplash, by Icons8 Team, 2018, https://unsplash.com/photos/NtwdMDylfTw/ Copyright 2018 by Icons8 Team/Unsplash.

Now, it's time to get practical. At this point, you would already have a strong motivation to start following the diet. As soon as you finish reading this book, you can apply everything you have learned to succeed on your OMAD journey. In this chapter, you will be learning everything else that you need to get started. As someone who has been following the OMAD method for some time now, I can tell you that it's totally achievable. I can also tell you that this eating pattern has benefited my life in so many ways. Now, let's prepare you to begin with the OMAD method of intermittent fasting...

START SLOW!

Since the OMAD method is quite extreme, the best way to approach it is by going slow. If it's your first time following intermittent fasting, then you may want to try one of the easier methods first. For instance, you can follow the 16:8 method for a few weeks or months just to help your body adjust and get familiar with fasting. Then you can make modifications to the method you have chosen by gradually increasing the length of your fasting window. To give you a more practical look at how your transition would go, here is an example of the steps you can follow:

- When you feel like you have adjusted to the first method that you are following, start increasing the duration of your fasts. For instance, if you follow the

16:8 method, increase your fasting window to 18 or 20 hours two to three times each week.
- When you feel more comfortable with longer fasts, you can start doing OMAD fasts one to two times a week.
- On Monday, you follow your modified 16:8 fasting method.
- On Tuesday, you follow the OMAD method, wherein you will eat a big meal that contains around 1,200 to 1,300 calories.
- On Wednesday, you have a regular eating day.
- On Thursday, you follow your modified 16:8 fasting method.
- On Friday, you follow the OMAD method, wherein you will eat a big meal that contains around 1,200 to 1,300 calories.
- On Saturday, you have a regular eating day.
- On Sunday, you follow your modified 16:8 fasting method.

This is just an example of how you can transition from your current IF method to OMAD. You can create your own plan and schedule to follow. As you are in the transition phase, don't forget to listen to your body and trust your instincts.

The plan and schedule you create depend on your starting point. For instance, if you have tried fasting in the past (not necessarily intermittent fasting) and you immediately want to try OMAD, then your plan would look different. The key here is to make sure that your health won't get compromised as you start following OMAD. For instance, if you have no fasting experience and you immediately follow the OMAD method every day for a whole week, you might experience a lot of adverse side effects. No matter what your health and fitness goals are, try not to rush through the process. Give yourself—and your body—time to adjust to intermittent fasting. This is true no matter what method you have chosen to follow. As long as you feel comfortable with your process and your body isn't stressed, then you're doing it correctly.

MEAL PLANNING FOR THE OMAD METHOD

Meal planning is a process where you take the time to sit down and plan your meals for a whole week. You can also plan your meals for a specific number of days. But the point is, meal planning is all about... planning your meals! If you already practice meal planning, you can still continue to do so while on OMAD. In fact, meal planning becomes easier when you follow this eating pattern. But if you haven't tried meal planning before, you may want to consider it. Meal planning helps make your life easier, simpler, and healthier.

If you plan to ease into OMAD, then your meal plans for the transition period might be a bit complex. After all, you would have to plan different numbers of meals for different days. For instance, going back to the example I shared in the last schedule, your meal plan for the week would look something like this:

- Monday (16:8): light breakfast, light lunch, and a light snack.
- Tuesday (OMAD): big breakfast.
- Wednesday (regular eating day): breakfast, lunch, snack, dinner.
- Thursday (16:8): light breakfast, light lunch, and a light snack.
- Friday (OMAD): big breakfast.
- Saturday (regular eating day): breakfast, lunch, snack, dinner.
- Sunday (16:8): light breakfast, light lunch, and a light snack.

You may follow this routine for a few weeks before making modifications to move you towards your goal of completely following the OMAD method. Each time you make modifications to your eating pattern, make sure to update your meal plan too. That way, you can shop for, prepare, and cook your meals accordingly. When making your meal plan for OMAD, here are some things for you to keep in mind:

- You aren't required to exclude any foods or food groups. However, it's best to avoid unhealthy foods as much as you can. You may have these indulgences once in a while—just not every day.

- Make sure that the meal you have planned will make you feel full and satisfied. While planning, remember that a lot of recipes are meant for single meal servings. Therefore, you have the option to eat more than a single serving of the dishes you cook or combine the dish with something else to increase the total number of calories.
- Take note of the macronutrient content of your meals. The macronutrients are protein, carbs, and fat. Also, try to make sure that each of your meals contains other essential vitamins, minerals, and nutrients. This will prevent you from developing a nutrient deficiency.
- If you want to be really healthy, focus on vegetables, fruits, high-quality lean proteins (organic, if possible), high-quality dairy products (organic, if possible), and complex carbs. You may also want to add healthy fats to your meals like olive oil and avocados to increase the nutritional value.
- If you don't think that you can eat enough to ensure that you're getting all of the nutrients your body requires to stay healthy, you may consider taking supplements. Before doing this, speak to your doctor first. Your doctor can give you advice on how to plan your meals better and what are the best supplements to take along with your OMAD eating pattern.

Meal planning helps you follow the OMAD method safely and effectively. When you plan your meals, you are also making sure that you're getting enough macro- and micronutrients for each of your meals. That way, you don't have to count your calories when it's time for you to eat. As long as you prepared or cooked the meal, you can also be sure that it is nutritious and filling enough.

If in the past, you had to think about 21 meals a week plus snacks, when you follow OMAD, your meal planning will go down to only seven meals a week. This means that you will save a lot of time and effort with this practical process. Let me share with you another example. This time, I will share a sample meal plan to give you an idea on what a week on OMAD will look like:

- Monday: Mac & cheese, roasted Brussels sprouts, and a turmeric ginger smoothie.
- Tuesday: Mexican-style tortilla soup with lentils, fresh fruit juice, and an apple muffin.
- Wednesday: Chickpea wraps, an avocado salad, and a mango smoothie.
- Thursday: Falafel sandwich with sweet potatoes, overnight oats, and fresh fruit juice.
- Friday: Quinoa power bowl, a piece of fruit, and an almond butter smoothie with blueberries.
- Saturday: Shepherd's pie, dinner rolls, and fruit juice.

- Sunday: Breakfast burritos, a side salad, and an avocado smoothie.

Most of the time, the meals you plan would contain a main meal, a side dish, a beverage, and a dessert if desired. For the rest of the day, continue to hydrate yourself with non-caloric beverages so you don't feel hungry all the time and you won't experience the common side effects of long periods of fasting. In the next section, there are more ideas for you to add to your meal plan. But this time, in the form of recipes.

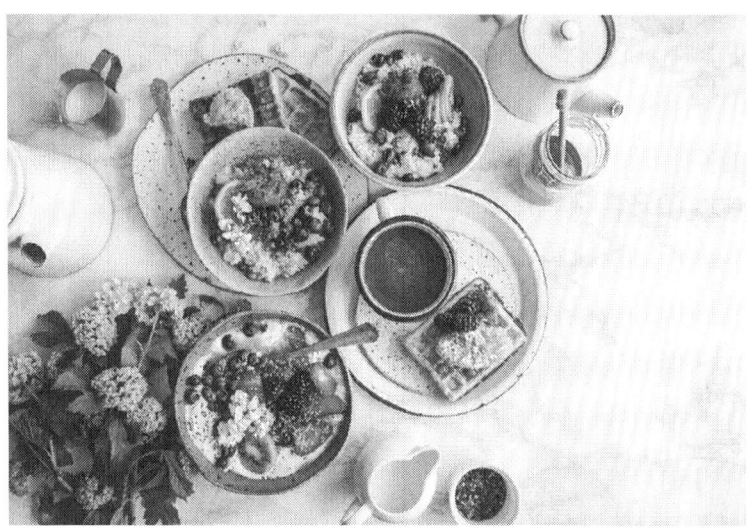

Fig. 8: Recipes. Unsplash, by Brooke Lark, 2017, https://unsplash.com/photos/HlNcigvUi4Q/ Copyright 2017 by Brooke Lark/Unsplash.

7 SUGGESTED RECIPES FOR YOUR OMAD METHOD MEAL PLANNING

Following the OMAD method doesn't have to be challenging. As long as you plan for it, you can ensure that you are getting enough calories each day to avoid compromising your health or developing any nutrient deficiencies. As much as possible, you should consume 1,200 calories on your single meal with the following macronutrient breakdown:

- Carbs: 10 grams
- Fat: 104 grams
- Protein: 105 grams

These are the ideal values, but you can practice flexibility so you won't have to be too strict when planning your meals. Here are a few recipes you can cook as you follow the OMAD method. These recipes are healthy, delicious, filling, and will provide you with the nutrients you need for the day.

Taco Bowl with Steak Strips

This is a low-carb recipe that's simple, healthy, and versatile too. You need only 20 minutes to create the whole dish, and you can even change up the ingredients as you see fit. For the steak strips, you can either cook them for this recipe or you can also use leftovers if you have any. Although this taco bowl requires simple ingredients, it packs a lot of flavors to make you feel satisfied with the single meal for the day.

Time: 20 minutes

Serving Size: 1 taco bowl

Prep Time: 10 minutes

Cook Time: 10 minutes

Nutritional Information:

- *Calories: 702 kcal*
- *Carbs: 8.8 grams*
- *Fat: 56.1 grams*
- *Protein: 34.3 grams*

Ingredients for the steak:

- 1 tsp lime juice (fresh)
- 1 tbsp ghee
- 2 tbsp cilantro (minced)
- ⅓ lb filet steak of your choice
- 1 cup of cauliflower rice (cooked)
- black pepper
- salt

Ingredients for the toppings:

- 1 tbsp sour cream
- ¼ cup of tomato salsa (homemade or store-bought)
- ½ jalapeño (sliced thinly)
- 1 small avocado (peeled, pitted, sliced)
- cilantro (optional, chopped, for garnish)
- 2 lemon wedges (optional, for garnish)

Directions:

- Pat the filet steak dry with a paper towel to remove excess moisture.
- Season the filet steak with salt and black pepper on all sides.
- In a skillet, add the ghee over medium-high heat.
- Add the seasoned filet steak to the skillet and sear on both sides for about 4 to 8 minutes. The cooking time depends on the level of doneness you prefer.
- Transfer the seared filet steak to a cutting board to rest.
- As the filet steak is resting, assemble the taco bowl. Start by adding the cauliflower rice, lime juice, and cilantro to a bowl then mix until well-combined.
- Add all of the topping ingredients and arrange as desired.
- Slice the filet steak into strips and add to the bowl. Garnish with cilantro and lemon wedges if using.
- Serve immediately.

You can also store the taco bowl for one day in the refrigerator. For this meal, you can either increase the quantities of the ingredients to reach the recommended number of calories or you can pair it with a side dish like a salad, a bowl of soup, or a cup of brown rice. A smoothie or a dessert like a peanut butter and banana muffin would be a great addition to this meal too.

Salmon Power Platter

While following the OMAD method, you don't have to create complex dishes for yourself. Here is another simple recipe where all you have to do is prepare all of the ingredients and bring them together in a single platter. This is a wholesome dish that bursts with flavor and nutrients. It also features salmon as the main ingredient, one of the healthiest foods out there. As with the previous recipe, you can also change, add, or replace the ingredients to suit your palate.

Time: 10 minutes

Serving Size: 2 platters (1 platter on OMAD)

Prep Time: 5 minutes

Cook Time: 5 minutes

Nutritional Information:

- *Calories: 537 kcal*
- *Carbs: 4.6 grams*

- *Fat: 39.9 grams*
- *Protein: 36 grams*

Ingredients for the bowl:

- 2 tsp water
- 2 tbsp pumpkin seeds
- 2 tbsp red onion (raw, chopped)
- ½ lb salmon fillet (cooked or smoked, flaked)
- ¼ cup of asparagus (chopped)
- 1 cup of salad greens (rinsed, drained)
- 1 medium avocado (peeled, pitted, sliced)
- 2 hard-boiled eggs (cut in half)

Ingredients for the dressing:

- 1 tsp horseradish
- ½ tbsp capers (finely chopped)
- 1 tbsp apple cider vinegar
- 1 tbsp olive oil
- 1 tbsp parsley (finely chopped)
- 2 tbsp mayonnaise
- black pepper
- salt

Directions:

- Make the dressing by combining all of the ingredients in a bowl. Mix well and set aside.
- After washing the salad greens, drain them on a salad spinner.
- In a microwaveable bowl, add the asparagus and water.
- Place the bowl in the microwave and cook the asparagus on high for about 3 to 6 minutes. The asparagus should have a vibrant green color while retaining the crunchy texture.
- Slice the salmon fillet into strips and place on a platter.
- Add the egg halves, avocado slices, onion, and the cooked asparagus then top with the salad greens.
- Sprinkle the pumpkin seeds all over the salad greens and drizzle with dressing.
- Serve immediately.

This recipe can make up to two servings but if you're on OMAD, you can have both servings for yourself. Then round off this rich and filling meal with a low-carb dessert like a flourless muffin or a low-carb mug cake.

Rainbow Bowl

While following the OMAD method, bowls and platters are the easiest, healthiest, and most filling options for you. This is because they contain several ingredients that you would simply have to bring together to create your meal. Bowl and platter meals are also very flexible allowing you to mix and match according to what you feel like eating for the day. This recipe allows you to "eat the rainbow" as it contains healthy ingredients of different colors.

Time: 25 minutes

Serving Size: 2 bowls (1 bowl on OMAD)

Prep Time: 5 minutes

Cook Time: 20 minutes

Nutritional Information:

- *Calories: 599 kcal*
- *Carbs: 63.6 grams*
- *Fat: 22.1 grams*
- *Protein: 39.5 grams*

Ingredients:

- ½ tsp cooking oil
- ½ tsp garlic powder
- ½ tsp onion powder
- 1 tsp kosher salt
- ½ tbsp cumin (ground)
- ½ tbsp oregano (dried)
- ½ tbsp sweet or hot smoked paprika
- ½ tbsp vegetable oil of your choice

- ¾ tbsp chili powder
- ½ lb ground beef (extra lean)
- ½ cup of corn (canned, drained)
- 1 cup of black beans (canned, rinsed, drained)
- 1 cup of cherry tomatoes (cut into halves)
- 1 cup of sweet potatoes (peeled, cubed)
- 1 small avocado (peeled, pitted, sliced)
- ½ tsp cayenne powder (optional)

Directions:

- Preheat your oven to 400° F.
- In a bowl, combine the garlic powder, salt, onion powder, cumin, oregano, paprika, and chili powder. Add cayenne pepper, if using, and mix everything together until well-combined.
- In a baking sheet, add the sweet potato cubes.
- Drizzle with vegetable oil and sprinkle half of the seasoning mixture.
- Toss the sweet potato cubes lightly until all pieces are evenly coated.
- Place the baking sheet in the oven and bake the sweet potato cubes for about 15 to 20 minutes until completely cooked through and tender.
- In the meantime, add cooking oil to a pan over medium heat.
- Once the oil is hot, add the ground beef and cook for

about 5 to 7 minutes. The ground beef must be completely cooked through. If excess oils are released from the ground beef, drain carefully. Just leave around 1 tablespoon of fat.
- Add the black beans to the pan along with the rest of the seasoning mixture.
- Toss the ingredients together until the ground beef and black beans are fully coated with oil and seasonings.
- Continue cooking until the beans are completely heated through. Keep tossing so that the ingredients won't stick to the pan.
- Add all of the ingredients in a bowl (the cooked and raw ingredients). Arrange as desired and serve immediately.

You can have both servings to yourself, and these would provide you with enough calories for the day. But you can also add more toppings like crumbled feta, jalapeños, sour cream, or green onion to make this bowl more flavorful. Then enjoy it with a refreshing glass of lemonade for a hearty, healthy meal.

Vegan Burritos

Burritos are very filling, especially when you use the right ingredients. This recipe offers a vegan twist to burritos, but you can also add some protein to it like steak slices, ground beef or shredded chicken. Doing this will add more calories to the dish, thus, bringing you closer to your daily caloric intake target. This is another easy recipe that comes together in just half an hour.

Time: 30 minutes

Serving Size: 2 burritos

Prep Time: 15 minutes

Cook Time: 15 minutes

Nutritional Information:

- *Calories: 713 kcal*
- *Carbs: 131 grams*
- *Fat: 14 grams*
- *Protein: 19 grams*

Ingredients for the filling:

- ¼ tsp chili powder
- ¼ tsp cumin
- ¼ tsp garlic powder
- 1 tbsp lime juice (fresh)
- 2 tbsp butter
- ¼ cup of cilantro (fresh, chopped)
- ¾ cup of rice (cooked)
- 1 cup of black beans (cooked with a pinch of salt, drained)

- 1 small red onion (sliced)
- 2 medium red potatoes (washed, peeled, cubed)
- black pepper
- sea salt

Ingredients for the slaw:

- 2 tbsp lime juice (fresh)
- 1 cup of purple cabbage (thinly sliced)
- ¼ medium avocado
- 1 jalapeño (seeds removed, sliced)
- black pepper
- sea salt

Ingredients for serving:

- ¼ cup of salsa (homemade or store-bought)
- ½ medium avocado (sliced)
- 2 large flour tortillas of your choice
- hot sauce of your choice (optional)

Directions:

- In a skillet, add the butter over medium heat and swirl around to coat the whole surface.
- Add the potato cubes on one side of the skillet and the

chopped onion on the other. Sprinkle with sea salt and black pepper.
- Cover the skillet and allow the vegetables to cook for about 4 to 5 minutes.
- Remove the cover, toss or flip the vegetables over, replace the cover, and continue cooking for about 4 to 5 minutes until golden brown.
- Remove the skillet from the heat then set aside.
- In a saucepan, add the beans over medium heat. Sprinkle with chili powder, garlic powder, and cumin.
- Mix the beans to coat them with the seasonings.
- When the beans release water and start bubbling, bring the heat down to low to keep the beans warm.
- In a bowl, add the avocado and mash. Add the lime juice and mix well.
- Add the jalapeño and cabbage then toss together to combine.
- Season with sea salt and black pepper, toss lightly, then set aside.
- Prepare the cooked rice by adding cilantro and lime juice. Use a fork to toss lightly.
- Warm the flour tortillas in the microwave for about 30 seconds. This will soften them too.
- Start assembling the tortillas. Add half of the rice to each tortilla.
- Continue adding the rest of the filling ingredients to the tortillas in any order.

- Top each of the tortillas with the avocado slaw, avocado slices, salsa, and hot sauce, if using.
- Wrap the burritos carefully and serve immediately.

If you have any leftover toppings, you can serve them on the side. You can have both burritos in one sitting but it might be too filling for you. Instead, you can store one of the burritos in the refrigerator and pair the other one with a filling side dish like a baked chicken breast or a pan-fried salmon fillet. You can also round off your meal with a decadent dessert like crème brulée or a slice of blueberry cheesecake.

Full-English Breakfast Plate

Here's a filling platter for you to enjoy at any time of the day. It's healthy, colorful, scrumptious, and oh-so-easy to bring together. Again, you can change some of the ingredients according to your preference. Just make sure that the ingredients you replace will help you reach your caloric intake target while adding variety to your meal. This tip applies to the other recipes too.

Time: 15 minutes

Serving Size: 1 plate

Prep Time: 5 minutes

Cook Time: 10 minutes

Nutritional Information:

- *Calories: 658 kcal*
- *Carbs: 7 grams*
- *Fat: 55 grams*
- *Protein: 29.6 grams*

Ingredients:

- 1 tbsp duck fat or ghee
- ½ cup of spinach (fresh, rinsed, drained)
- 1 small avocado (peeled, pitted, sliced)
- 2 large eggs
- 2 to 3 slices of bacon
- 5 to 6 brown mushrooms
- 5 to 6 cherry tomatoes (still on the vine)
- black pepper
- salt
- chili pepper flakes (optional)
- 2 Italian sausages (optional, for added protein)

Directions:

- In a skillet, add the duck fat over medium-high heat.
- Add the mushrooms with their top side-down.
- Season with salt and black pepper then cook for about 5 minutes.

- Flip the mushrooms over and continue cooking for about 2 minutes until tender.
- Take the cooked mushrooms out of the skillet and set aside.
- In a pan, fry the bacon over medium heat until your desired level of doneness.
- Once cooked, place on a paper towel to drain excess oils.
- In the same pan, fry the eggs according to your preference.
- Once cooked, transfer to your serving plate.
- Turn up the heat to high, add the vine of cherry tomatoes, and cook for about 1 minute. If you want to serve the tomatoes raw, you can skip this step.
- If you want to add Italian sausages to your platter, cook them on the same pan too.
- Add all of the ingredients (cooked and raw) to the serving platter along with the eggs. Arrange them as desired.
- Top with avocado slices and serve immediately.

This amazing dish bursts with different flavors and textures. On its own, it's quite filling already. But you can also pair it with a thick and creamy bowl of roasted squash soup or a decadent dessert like apple pie a la mode.

Warm and Rich Coconut Curry

This recipe is simple, packed with veggies, and full of flavors. It's a definite crowd-pleaser that's gluten-free and vegan too. Although this is one of the lighter options I will share with you, it's great on OMAD because you can pair it with different side dishes to create a hearty, healthy meal for the day.

Time: 30 minutes

Serving Size: 2 bowls (1 bowl for OMAD)

Prep Time: 5 minutes

Cook Time: 25 minutes

Nutritional Information:

- *Calories: 434 kcal*
- *Carbs: 41 grams*
- *Fat: 25.8 grams*
- *Protein: 10.2 grams*

Ingredients:

- ½ tbsp curry powder
- ½ tbsp ginger (fresh, grated)
- ½ tbsp olive oil
- ⅛ cup of snow peas (sliced in half)
- ⅛ cup of tomatoes (diced)
- ¼ cup of broccoli florets (diced)

- ¼ cup of carrots (diced)
- ½ cup of vegetable broth (homemade or store-bought)
- 1 cup of coconut quinoa (cooked using 1 ¾ cup of coconut milk)
- 1 ¾ cup of coconut milk
- 1 small onion (diced)
- 2 cloves of garlic (minced)
- black pepper
- sea salt
- ½ tsp cayenne powder (optional, for cooking)
- ½ tsp red pepper flakes (optional, for serving)
- 2 lemon wedges (optional, for serving)

Directions:

- Start by cooking the coconut quinoa.
- In a pot, add the coconut oil over medium heat.
- Add the garlic, onion, carrots, broccoli florets, ginger, sea salt, and black pepper then stir to combine.
- Cook the vegetables for about 5 minutes until softened. Stir frequently so the vegetables don't stick to the bottom of the pot.
- Add the coconut milk, vegetable broth, curry powder, salt, black pepper, and cayenne powder if using.
- Mix the ingredients together and bring to a boil.
- Once boiling, lower the heat slightly, and simmer for about 10 to 15 minutes. While cooking, taste the

- mixture and add more seasonings according to your preference.
- In the last 5 minutes of cooking, add the tomatoes and snow peas.
- Pour the curry into a bowl and garnish with lemon wedges and red pepper, if using.
- Serve immediately with coconut quinoa.

Note: To cook the coconut quinoa, add ½ tablespoon of cooking oil to a saucepan over medium heat. Add 1 cup of quinoa and cook for about 5 minutes until golden. Stir often so it doesn't burn. Add 1½ cups of water, 1 ¾ cups of coconut milk, and a pinch of salt then mix well. Bring the mixture to a boil and turn the heat down to low. Cover the saucepan and allow to simmer for about 20 to 25 minutes until all of the liquid has evaporated and the quinoa is cooked. Use a fork to fluff and set aside while you prepare the curry dish.

If you will eat both servings, then you can round off your meal with a decadent dessert like a chocolate lava cake. But if you will only have one bowl of this curry with half of the coconut quinoa, then you can complete your meal with some kind of protein like grilled chicken or a baked fillet of fish.

Pan-Fried Pork Chop with Hollandaise Sauce and Asparagus

This last dish would be perfect for an easy and quick weeknight dinner. It's the perfect combination of sweet asparagus, tender pork chops, and a lovely hollandaise sauce that ties all the flavors together. You can even use the sauce for other dishes once you've learned how to make it.

Time: 35 minutes

Serving Size: 1 serving

Prep Time: 10 minutes

Cook Time: 25 minutes

Nutritional Information:

- *Calories: 690 kcal*
- *Carbs: 2.8 grams*
- *Fat: 58.8 grams*
- *Protein: 36 grams*

Ingredients:

- 1 tbsp ghee
- 1 tbsp lemon juice (fresh)
- ½ cup of butter (melted)
- ¾ cup of asparagus spears
- 1 pork loin chop (bone-in)
- 3 large eggs (yolks only)
- salt
- black pepper

Directions:

- Start by preparing the hollandaise sauce first. In a jar with a wide mouth, add the butter. The mouth of the jar should be wide enough so that you can fit a hand blender into it. If you don't have such a jar, make the sauce in a microwaveable bowl first then transfer into a jar.
- Add the lemon juice and egg yolks in the butter, then blend with a hand blender.
- As you're blending, lift the hand blender slowly. Taste the sauce and add salt and black pepper according to your preference. Set the sauce aside.
- Add the ghee in a pan over medium-high heat.
- Add the pork chop to the pan and cook one side for about 6 minutes.
- Flip the pork chop over and continue cooking the other side for another 6 minutes.
- Take the pork chop out of the pan and allow it to rest for about 5 minutes.
- In a pot, add water (enough to submerge the asparagus spears), and bring to a boil.
- Once boiling, add the asparagus spears and blanch for about 5 minutes.
- Take the asparagus spears out of the water. Drain well.
- On a plate, add the pork chop and the asparagus spears on the side.

- Drizzle with the homemade hollandaise sauce and serve.

Since this recipe calls for the use of raw eggs, you may opt for pasteurized eggs to be on the safer side. Store the rest of the sauce in the refrigerator for up to 4 days with an airtight lid. Warm it a bit before use. You can make this meal more filling by having a cup of rice with it or a thick, hearty soup. If not, you can also end the meal with an indulgent dessert like a soufflé.

OTHER ESSENTIAL TIPS

Although intermittent fasting, specifically the OMAD method isn't a diet, it still involves making changes in your eating habits. I have already shared with you some of the most practical guidelines for following this eating pattern. Now, let us go through a few essential tips to increase your chances of following this extreme IF method:

1. Make sure that you are properly hydrated throughout the day

At one time each day, you will enjoy your full, healthy meal. Before and after that meal, you can still consume non-caloric beverages to ensure that you don't get dehydrated. Some examples of non-caloric beverages are plain coffee, tea, and, of course, water. Maintaining proper hydration is essential, especially if you want to lose weight on OMAD. If you feel hungry at any point before or after your meal, drinking the recommended beverages can help you control your hunger pangs and cravings. The longer you follow OMAD, the more you will notice that your cravings and hunger pangs are diminishing too.

Here's a practical tip for you in terms of hydration—drinking a glass of sparkling water with fresh lemon or lime juice in the morning can help boost your electrolyte levels. OMAD tends to throw off your electrolyte levels, thus, it is important to replenish your electrolytes to ensure your health. You can also add magnesium powder or salt to a glass of water to achieve the same effect. Also, it's more effective to have this glass of water in the morning.

2. Learn how to cook your meals so that you can enjoy a wide variety of dishes

One of the best benefits of meal planning is that it allows you to diversify your diet to keep it interesting. You might think that OMAD will trigger food cravings, and if you eat the same thing each day, you will probably get bored with this eating pattern. On the other hand, if you vary your foods each day, you can make this extreme IF method more interesting, fulfilling, and motivating.

Aside from meal planning, cooking your own meals also allows you to change things up. Cooking can be a very relaxing hobby. When you gain confidence in your cooking skills, you can start looking for more exotic recipes to excite your taste buds. Basically, indulging in a wide variety of foods makes it easier to follow OMAD or any other intermittent fasting method.

3. Eat foods from different food groups

Since you will only be eating once a day, make sure that your plate is filled with foods from different food groups. For instance, if you love eating steaks, it's not the best idea to simply eat one big steak a day and nothing else. Instead, you can have different kinds of steaks that you would pair with a side of buttered vegetables, a light salad, mashed potatoes, or a bowl of soup. This variety makes it easier for you to consume all of the nutrients your body needs each day.

Speaking of steaks, while following OMAD, your plate should always contain a source of protein. Biologically speaking, protein is the most important nutrient you should have. Aside from being good for your health, protein is also filling. Therefore, a meal with a good protein source can help tide you over until the next day when it's time for you to eat your next meal.

4. Stay productive while following the OMAD method

One of the benefits of the OMAD method is better concentration and focus. As these improve, so will your productivity. Take advantage of this benefit by trying to stay productive throughout the day. Staying productive offers two advantages. First, you will have the chance to do everything you need to accomplish for the day. For instance, if you are swamped at work, you will have the time (along with focus and concentration) to accomplish everything without having to think about when or what you will eat during your break time.

The second benefit of staying productive is it can help distract you from the hunger you feel. This is especially helpful at the beginning of your OMAD journey when you are likely to feel hunger or cravings. If you're distracted or busy with your tasks at home or at work, you won't be thinking about your hunger or the fact that your next meal is still hours away.

5. Learn how to relax and make sure that you're always getting enough sleep

At some point, you might feel like OMAD is taking a toll on your health. Since you will be restricting your calories through your eating pattern, you have to make sure that all the other aspects of your life are taken care of too. Relaxation can help make things a lot easier for you. If you feel stressed because you think that you cannot make it to your next meal, try performing relaxation techniques like taking a long soak in the bathtub with a cup of tea or meditation, for example. These activities will help you overcome such feelings. Of course, if they don't go away and you can't focus on anything else, you can give in and allow yourself to eat a light snack. You may have to do this a few times in the beginning.

Getting enough sleep is also essential to your health. Think about it: if you follow an extreme eating pattern like OMAD

PREPARING TO FOLLOW THE OMAD METHOD OF INT... | 115

and you get only three or four hours of sleep each night, you might end up getting ill. You will experience fatigue, dizziness, and other common side effects. But if you make sure that you get enough sleep each night, you are also giving your body a chance to repair and refresh itself for the next day.

6. Engage in light exercises

If you work out regularly, you don't have to stop while following the OMAD diet. However, you may want to decrease the intensity of your workouts, especially when you're starting out. But if you're used to high-intensity workouts, make sure to have your one meal of the day after your workout session. This ensures that you replenish the resources you lost while working out.

If you plan to ease into the OMAD method, then it's recommended to work out on days when you are not scheduled to follow OMAD. For instance, in the example I shared in the meal planning section, the OMAD days are on Tuesday and Friday. This means that you can work out on Monday, Wednesday, Thursday, Saturday, and Sunday. It's all about planning your schedule and your exercise activities to make sure that neither your health nor your workout routine gets compromised.

7. Consider using an app to help you out

These days, there are apps for virtually anything—even for following OMAD. One example of such an app is Cronometer. This app helps you make sure that you are always meeting your recommended daily requirements as you follow the OMAD method. With this app, you can keep track of your calories, log the meals you eat, add notes, create custom foods, and more. If you think that you need all the help you can get to succeed on this diet, then apps like Cronometer can help you out.

8. Change things up once in a while

Finally, it would be more beneficial for you to change your eating pattern once in a while. Although OMAD is highly effective and easy to follow, changing up your method once in a while prevents metabolic adaptation. The changes will keep your body guessing so that you don't have to worry about your metabolism slowing down because it's too used to being "starved." Changing your eating pattern once in a while is the smarter and more sustainable way to approach OMAD.

As you can see, all of these tips are practical, easy, and effective. Although you don't have to follow these tips (and the ones I shared earlier), keeping them in mind while you follow OMAD will help improve your chances of experiencing benefits from it. Of course, you should also know if this eating pattern is no longer working for you.

WHEN TO STOP

The OMAD diet isn't for everyone—I cannot stress this enough. Although it works well for me and for every other proponent of the OMAD method, it might not work for you. Although you might feel disappointed about this, you should still know when to stop. For one, if OMAD is making you sick, stop. If you are suffering from a medical condition and it is getting worse because of OMAD, stop. If you consult with your doctor and they tell you that this eating pattern isn't suitable for you, listen to your doctor. Although OMAD can potentially change your life for the better, if it isn't happening for you, know when to stop. Your health and safety should always be your priority. If OMAD isn't right for you, give the other methods a try.

This is why you should learn how to listen to your body—so that you can determine whether you can continue with OMAD or you should discontinue it. This method might not be alright for you and that's okay. Intermittent fasting can be done in different ways. Maybe another method would work better for you. Or maybe you just need more time for your body to adjust. After following a different method for some time, then you may consider giving OMAD a try again. It's also important for you to be aware of the potential risks and side effects of the OMAD method. This awareness will help you make better choices as you follow the eating pattern or if you choose to stop.

6

THE POTENTIAL RISKS AND SIDE EFFECTS OF THE OMAD METHOD

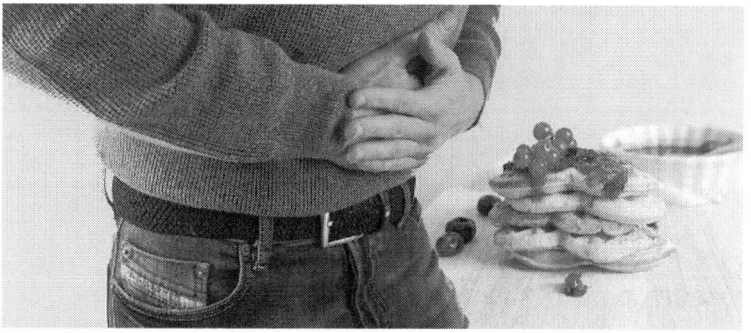

Fig. 9: Hunger. Pixabay, by mohamed Hassan, 2018, https://pixabay.com/photos/stomach-health-diet-dessert-eating-3532098/ Copyright 2018 by mohamed Hassan/Unsplash.

At this point, you have almost everything you need to start following the OMAD method. But I want to share with you all of the essential aspects of this eating pattern for you to make an informed decision on whether to follow it or not.

This means that I will also be sharing with you the "other side of the coin."

While there might be a lot of resources about OMAD online, most of them only have a single focus. Some only focus on the good sides while some only focus on the bad sides. If you only look at the good side of OMAD, you might start following the eating pattern without knowing what to expect or what to avoid. On the other hand, if you only focus on the bad side of OMAD, then you probably won't even bother learning more. This means that you would have wasted an opportunity to make a positive change in your life.

Now that I have shared with you all of the good things to expect from the OMAD method, it's time to learn the potential risks and side effects. Then you can decide whether this method is right for you or if you want to try other methods first.

THE RISKS OF OMAD AND OTHER INTERMITTENT FASTING METHODS

Just like any other extreme diet or eating plan, OMAD comes with its own set of risks. Beneficial as it is, it can also pose dangers to your health, which is why I keep reminding you that this eating method isn't for everyone. But if you are aware of these risks, you might have a better chance of avoiding them. Also, knowing the potential risks of OMAD allows you to recognize them as soon as they start happening to you. As you consider following OMAD or while you are following this eating pattern, look out for these risks:

1. You will experience hunger pangs like never before

This is one of the most common risks of the OMAD method. Eating once a day is very different from eating three times a day, plus having one or two snacks in between. Naturally, when you start fasting, then you will experience frequent hunger pangs. These, in turn, can lead to cravings. Once you give in to your cravings, then you might develop a problematic relationship with food. Even if you can get through your hunger pangs, you might end up binge eating on every meal. Even if you only have one meal a day, this can be very troublesome for you if you binge every day.

If you want to overcome this issue or avoid this risk, expect to experience hunger. Since you will be skipping meals and only eating a single meal each day, the natural response of your body is to feel hungry. As much as possible, try to resist the urge to eat. You can distract yourself with different activities, drink some kind of non-caloric beverage or do anything else that will help take your mind off your hunger. However, if you feel like you cannot control your hunger anymore and it's starting to take a toll on you, then you can eat something light and healthy to tide you over. Remember—you should never compromise your health and well-being.

If you discover that this eating pattern is causing you to binge eat every day, then you may want to re-think your decision to follow the OMAD method. Maybe give yourself more time to adjust to fasting by following a different method first. After your body has adjusted to an easier IF method, then you can try following OMAD again. Hopefully, this time, you can handle your hunger and cravings better.

2. You could get dehydrated if you don't drink enough water

One of the tips I have shared with you in the previous chapters is to keep drinking water and other non-caloric beverages throughout your fasting window. This is very important so that you don't end up getting dehydrated while fasting. This is especially important if you lead an active lifestyle or you are doing a lot of things during your fasting window. Dehydration is very serious, so you must avoid this at all costs. Fortunately, this risk is easier to avoid. All you have to do is be conscious of your liquid intake. No matter how busy you are, make sure that you're drinking enough to keep you hydrated throughout the day.

3. You may experience fatigue, tiredness, and difficulty concentrating

These risks are quite common, especially at the beginning. Since you will be reducing your caloric intake significantly, you would be at risk of experiencing these symptoms. To avoid any issues, easing into the OMAD method is key. Then you can schedule this method on days when you don't have a lot of work or physical activity to do. During your fasting window, you can perform relaxing activities to take your mind off your hunger while avoiding fatigue, tiredness, and difficulty concentrating.

4. You could develop nutritional deficiencies

This is one of the more dangerous risks of the OMAD method. Again, it can come from the caloric restriction that you would be imposing on yourself because you would only be eating one meal each day. You can avoid this risk by making sure that each meal you consume contains a healthy balance of vegetables, fruits, proteins, healthy fats, and complex carbohydrates. Even though you are technically allowed to eat anything you want while on OMAD, it's still recommended to focus on healthy, whole foods to ensure that you won't develop nutrient deficiencies.

Go to your doctor regularly to have your nutrient levels checked. If you find out that you are lacking in specific nutrients, increase your intake of foods that contain those nutrients. Otherwise, you may consider taking supplements after asking your doctor if this is the right step to take.

5. You may experience appetite deregulation

When you shift to OMAD or any other IF method, your appetite changes. In the past, your body would already have an idea of when it's time to eat because you have been following the same eating pattern every day. As you transition into intermittent fasting, you may notice that your appetite isn't the same as it was in the past. While this might not be considered much of a risk to some people, appetite deregulation may also have an effect on your mood.

The reason for this is that the part of the brain that regulates the appetite is the same part of the brain that regulates mood. When nutrient consumption is affected, and appetite deregulation happens, you might experience changes in your mood too. One of the most common changes is irritability—and you might experience this while you are fasting. For this risk, the best thing you can do is try to eat healthily. That way, your body won't suffer because of a lack of nutrients. You can also try relaxation techniques to help make you feel better while you are fasting.

6. Your metabolism might slow down

Finally, if you follow OMAD long term, your metabolism might start slowing down. It won't work efficiently simply because it doesn't have to. Then when you shift back to a normal diet, you might gain a lot of weight. This is why it's recommended to change your method once in a while. That way, your body won't get used to OMAD so much that the slowing down becomes a permanent effect.

These are the most common risks of the OMAD diet. I have also shared some tips on how to avoid them. As long as you are aware of the changes happening to your body and you always listen to your body, there is a good chance that you can avoid these risks. However, if you think that these risks are too much for you to handle, then you may want to come up with your own plan for how to deal with and overcome them if you still want to follow the OMAD method.

SIGNS THAT THE OMAD METHOD ISN'T FOR YOU

The potential risks of the OMAD method aren't the only things to be aware of when you start following it. A lot of us have thrived while following this method but for some people, they realize at some point that OMAD isn't right for them. In such a case, you can either change your approach to the eating pattern or find another method to follow. Either way, if you experience the following signs, it might mean that OMAD isn't the best lifestyle choice for you. Just like being aware of the risks so that you can recognize them when they happen, it's important to look out for these signs that you and OMAD aren't a good fit:

1. If you start becoming obsessed with food

As I had been successful in my own OMAD journey, I can tell you that over time, it gets easier. In the beginning, I was always thinking about my next meal: when I would have it, what I would eat, and how many more hours I would have to wait before I can enjoy another big meal. As the weeks went by, I learned how to distract myself by doing more productive things. I also made sure to hydrate myself throughout the day, so I wouldn't have to think about the hunger I was feeling. Without even realizing it, I had already stopped focusing on my one meal of the day. It became part of my routine.

But when you start becoming obsessed with food, that's a different story. For some people, once they finish their one meal of the day, they feel satisfied. But after a while, their thoughts go back to the food they ate. Then they start feeling overly concerned about what their next meal will be and when they can eat again. If you experience this, it can be an indicator that the OMAD method isn't for you. The main problem with developing an obsession with food is that it may lead to an eating disorder. So if you can't stop thinking about food and it's starting to take over your life, you may have to rethink your choice.

2. If you start feeling guilty about eating

Eating is a natural thing. In fact, it's a necessity. So when you eat your one meal of the day, you should enjoy and relish the experience. After all, this meal is meant to nourish your body and keep you healthy. Since you will only be eating one meal a day, then the meal would be substantially bigger than what you're used to. However, if you feel guilty about consuming so much—even when you know that this is the only meal you will have for the day—then the OMAD method becomes a negative experience for you.

Feelings of guilt or even self-shaming are never good for your well-being. As you transition into OMAD, learn how to be kind to yourself. If you can't stick with the eating pattern rigidly, forgive yourself. Don't berate yourself for giving in to your hunger and eating a light snack. But if the negative feelings don't go away no matter how much you try to convince yourself to be kinder, then this might be another indication that OMAD isn't right for you.

3. When you feel excessive levels of stress

Intermittent fasting tends to increase your cortisol levels. Since OMAD is an extreme method of IF, this means that you might experience high levels of this hormone, which, in turn, makes you feel excessive levels of stress. While OMAD potentially offers a lot of health benefits, if it makes you too stressed to function normally, then this eating pattern might not be the best choice for you to make right now. Before giving up, give relaxation techniques a try. If they work, good for you! You can keep going. But if they don't, then you may have to try other methods of fasting intermittently.

4. When you frequently feel "hangry"

Have you ever felt hangry before? This occurs when you feel so hungry that virtually anything can set you off. A lot of people who start diets or embark on new eating patterns may experience feeling hangry. This is normal. But, again, if you are on OMAD and you notice that you're always hangry, it's time to make a change. Think about it: if you follow OMAD every day, this means that you will feel hangry every day too. Do you really want this feeling to be part of your life? If not, then you may want to find a different method—one that doesn't make you feel hangry all the time.

5. When you feel like "something is off"

If you learn how to listen to your body, you will know what it feels like to be healthy, and you will also know if something's wrong. As you follow OMAD, it's important to listen to your body's cues by increasing your awareness. If you feel like your health is declining and you aren't getting all the nutrients you need to stay healthy, it's time to make a change. You may try modifying your one meal of the day first. Opt for healthier and more diverse foods. You may even increase your caloric intake a bit. But if these changes don't improve the way you feel, if you still feel like something's off, then OMAD might not be for you.

6. When you cannot sleep well

For some people, OMAD might be causing such big changes in their bodies that they start experiencing sleep disturbances like insomnia. Such effects are a huge no-no since sleep is critical to your health. No matter what diet or eating pattern you are following, getting enough sleep every night should be part of the equation. But if fasting is causing issues with your sleeping patterns, then maybe you should try something else.

If you experience any of these signs, don't give up right away. Remember that OMAD is a flexible method just like all the other IF methods available. Consider your approach first and try making a few changes. If the changes you make solve your issue, then you can continue following OMAD. But if you still experience these issues no matter how many times you have tweaked your approach to the OMAD method, then you can make the choice to start following a different IF method.

In such a case, you must already have an exit strategy. Although you want to succeed on OMAD, having a plan to transition out of this method is a wise thing. Even if you succeed, you might choose to go back to your old eating habits after some time. When you reach this point, then you would need your exit strategy too. This will make it easier for you to go back to your old eating patterns without worrying that all of the benefits will go away. It's all about learning how to use your diet and eating patterns to your advantage so that you can achieve your long-term health goals.

WHO SHOULDN'T FOLLOW INTERMITTENT FASTING?

In general, intermittent fasting isn't a good fit for everyone. Whether you choose OMAD or any other method of intermittent fasting, you will be making a commitment to changing your eating pattern in a big way. If you decide to skip meals once in a while just because you're not hungry, you can't really say that you're following IF. While spontaneous meal skipping can be a way for you to start on IF, committing to any of the IF methods is a different thing.

Intermittent fasting offers a number of benefits. However, there are certain groups of people who shouldn't be following this eating pattern. In this last section, we will be going through the different groups of people who should follow IF, those who should consider it very carefully, and those who shouldn't even attempt to follow the diet. Try to see which group you fall under so that you can decide whether it's time for you to follow IF or if you need to make any other preparations before you start, especially if you're planning to follow OMAD.

People who can follow intermittent fasting freely

Generally, there are people who have a higher likelihood of succeeding in IF. Although I didn't technically fall into any of these categories, I had the drive and commitment to follow this trendy eating pattern. I also made sure that I learned everything I can about IF before following it. You can follow IF freely if you:

- Have tried dieting before.
- Have experience monitoring your caloric intake.
- Are healthy and you have a regular workout routine.
- Have a job that allows you to make changes in your eating patterns even if it means having to undergo the potential effects of the transition period.

- Are single or you live alone.
- Don't have any children.
- Have a partner who follows IF or if your partner is open and supportive of your dietary decisions.
- You're a man.

If you fall into any of these categories, then starting on IF might be easier for you. However, even if you're at the peak of health, it's still recommended to talk to your doctor first before you start on IF. You can even have a blood test to check if you have any issues that you don't know about. These steps can give you more confidence in yourself to start following intermittent fasting.

People who should consider this lifestyle change carefully first

If you don't fall into any of the previous categories, then you may want to proceed with caution when it comes to intermittent fasting. If you belong to the following categories, think about this change in lifestyle first and come up with a plan before you start:

- Your job requires you to be at your highest performance all the time. This might make it difficult for you to transition into OMAD.
- You are married, you have children or you live with other people in your home. It might be challenging to

stick with fasting when the rest of your family eat all throughout the day.
- You are an athlete, you compete in sports or you have a strict training regimen. In such a case, you may want to check with your coach or doctor first to ensure that your performance won't get compromised.
- You're a woman. Remember that women should be more cautious when approaching IF.

If you fall into any of these categories, this doesn't mean that you shouldn't follow intermittent fasting. It just means that you should be more careful if you decide to start fasting intermittently. Check with your doctor, educate yourself, and come up with a plan for IF to increase your chances of success.

PEOPLE WHO SHOULDN'T FOLLOW INTERMITTENT FASTING

Finally, there are certain groups of people who shouldn't try intermittent fasting at all. If you fall into any of these categories, try to think of other ways to improve your health. Otherwise, try to improve or change your situation first before you even consider going on IF. It's not recommended for you to follow intermittent fasting if:

You're pregnant or breastfeeding

If you're pregnant or breastfeeding, you need extra energy, thus, you shouldn't be fasting. If you're pregnant, fasting might have adverse effects on the developing fetus in your womb. If you're breastfeeding, you might not have enough nutrients to produce milk for your baby. So it's best to wait until your little one is old enough before you should consider following IF.

You're chronically stressed

Remember that IF can cause you to feel stressed. If you already suffer from chronic stress, going on IF might exacerbate your condition. Learn how to manage your stress better first before you try fasting intermittently.

You have never tried dieting, fasting or exercising before

Although IF can help you lose weight, it's not a good idea for you to follow this eating pattern if you have never tried following a diet, you never exercise or you have never experienced fasting before. Try to prepare your body for intermittent fasting first by developing a workout routine. Then you can also try skipping meals once in a while so you can experience what it feels like to fast. Whatever you do, don't try to jump into IF right away as it might do more harm to your health than good.

You have a history of or you are currently suffering from an eating disorder

Intermittent fasting can make you feel like you're struggling with food. This, in turn, might re-awaken your bad relationship with food, thus, causing more problems for you. Even if you had successfully overcome an eating disorder, you might be at risk for it recurring if you follow intermittent fasting.

You suffer from type 1 diabetes

Although IF can be beneficial for people who suffer from type 2 diabetes, it might not be the best option for those who suffer from type 1 diabetes. This is mainly because you won't be eating meals regularly. If you suffer from this condition and you really want to follow IF, even the simplest method, consult with your doctor and the rest of your health care team first.

OTHER PEOPLE WHO SHOULDN'T FOLLOW IF

- Women trying to conceive.
- Children and teenagers.
- People who suffer from kidney problems.
- People who suffer from adrenal problems.
- People who are underweight.
- People who are taking medications that require regular consumption of meals.
- People who already have sleeping disturbances.

If you fall under any of these categories, then you may want to consider another dietary approach to improve your health. Of course, if you can improve your current situation then you may consider IF sometime in the future. It's also not recommended to start fasting intermittently if this eating pattern doesn't fit into your lifestyle or routine. Now that you know pretty much everything about IF, specifically about the OMAD method, you should already have a good idea of whether this is the right path for you to take or not.

One last thing I would like to say in favor of intermittent fasting is the benefit of customization. Unlike diets, intermittent fasting allows you to customize the method you choose according to your needs. This is one of the most important reasons why so many people succeed on this diet. If you really want to give it a try, don't forget this aspect of the diet. Keep making changes while keeping the basic concept of the method you have chosen until you find the perfect way for you to live comfortably while following intermittent fasting.

CONCLUSION: YOUR INTERMITTENT FASTING JOURNEY

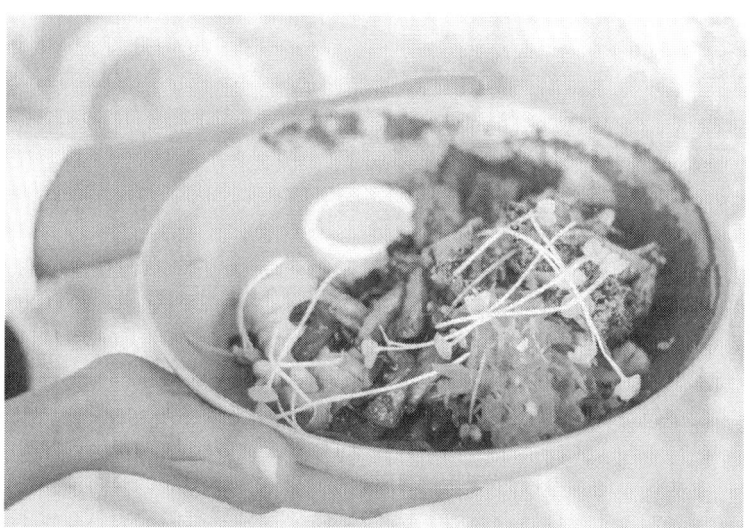

Fig. 10: Starting OMAD. Unsplash, by Maddi Bazzocco, 2018, https://unsplash.com/photos/qKbHvzXb85A/ Copyright 2018 by Maddi Bazzocco/Unsplash.

The OMAD method of intermittent fasting can potentially put you on a clearer path to health, happiness, and longevity. From start to finish, you have learned everything you need to know about the OMAD method—both good and bad—to determine whether it's right for you or not. If you decide to follow this method for the improvement of your health, then all you have to do is take that all-important first step.

In this book, we started off by learning all about intermittent fasting. As I have explained, this global trend isn't actually a diet. It's an eating pattern. Therefore, your focus won't be on the foods you will eat, but the time when you will eat your meals. It seems so simple and easy, but the more you learn about it, the more you realize how amazing intermittent fasting really is. To help you understand how and why this eating pattern works so well, we discussed what happens to your body when you eat and when you fast. The benefits of this eating pattern come during your fasting windows, the time when you aren't eating anything.

Speaking of benefits, we discussed all of the wonderful benefits of intermittent fasting in Chapter 2. As you have learned, this simple eating pattern offers a number of benefits to your health. If you can follow it correctly and stick with it long-term, IF can bring a lot of positive changes to your life. In Chapter 3, we discussed the most common methods of intermittent fasting. Although this eBook is focused on OMAD, learning about the other methods, and how to follow them can help you in your journey. This is especially true if you plan to start with a simpler method first before following OMAD.

In the next chapter, we started focusing on the One Meal A Day or OMAD method. Here, we defined what OMAD is and how to follow it. We also discussed the benefits of this specific method along with some initial tips for how to follow this extreme eating pattern. Here, I also introduced some of the downsides of OMAD, the other side that you should also know about so that you can truly determine if it is right for you. In Chapter 5, you were introduced to practical information about following the OMAD method. From starting slow, planning your meals, more tips, and knowing when to stop, this chapter should help you start your OMAD journey right away. It is in this chapter where I also shared a number of recipes for you to try out.

In the last chapter, we focused on the "dark side" of OMAD. Just like any other diet or eating pattern, OMAD also comes with its own risks. After all, it is one of the more extreme methods of intermittent fasting. If you think that you can follow OMAD without experiencing these side effects and risks, then it's time for you to begin. As I had promised you at the beginning of this book, I have shared everything I've learned as I embarked on my own OMAD journey. I started out wanting to overcome my insulin sensitivity and now, I have done that—and more.

As my final piece of advice for you, just remember to always listen to your body. If you think that you can succeed on OMAD while putting your health and safety first, then there is a very high chance that you will succeed. Thank you so much for taking the time to learn all about the OMAD method of intermittent fasting and how it can benefit your health. Now, as you finish this eBook, I wish you all the best on your OMAD journey. Hopefully, you will join us as one of the proponents of this extreme yet, highly beneficial eating pattern.

DOWNLOAD YOUR FREE CHEAT SHEET

(<u>Don't</u> start fasting before you've consulted this cheat sheet...)

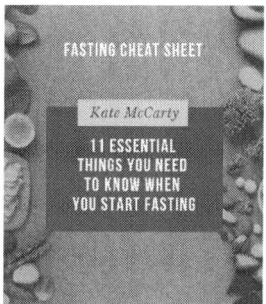

This cheat sheet includes:

- 11 things to know and to do while you are fasting.
- Why you need to know those things to start successfully.
- These things will make the process easier and more enjoyable.

The last thing I want is that the fasting process will be uncomfortable.

To receive your fasting cheat sheet, scan this QR code:

REFERENCES

30-Minute Coconut Curry. (n.d.). Retrieved from https://minimalistbaker.com/30-minute-coconut-curry/#_a5y_p=1531167

Allaf, M., Elghazaly, H., Mohamed, O. G., Fareen, F. K., Zaman, S., Salmasi, A. M., ... Dehghan, A. (2019). Intermittent fasting for the prevention of cardiovascular disease. Retrieved from https://www.cochranelibrary.com/cdsr/doi/10.1002/14651858.CD013496/full

Anton, S. D., Moehl, K., Donahoo, W., & Marosi, K. (2017). Flipping the Metabolic Switch: Understanding and Applying the Health Benefits of Fasting: Flipping the Metabolic Switch. Retrieved from https://www.researchgate.net/publication/320733870_Flipping_the_Metabolic_Switch_Under

standing_and_Applying_the_Health_Benefits_of_Fasting_Flipping_the_Metabolic_Switch

Antoni, R., Johnston, K. L., Collins, A. L., & Robertson, M. D. (2014). The Effects of Intermittent Energy Restriction on Indices of Cardiometabolic Health. Retrieved from https://ibimapublishing.com/articles/ENDO/2014/459119/

Antunes, F., Erustes, A. G., Costa, A. J., Nascimento, A. C., Bincoletto, C., Ureshino, R. P., ... Smaili, S. S. (2018). Autophagy and intermittent fasting: the connection for cancer therapy? Retrieved from https://www.ncbi.nlm.nih.gov/pmc/articles/PMC6257056/

Arnason, T. G., Bowen, M. W., & Mansell, K. D. (2017). Effects of intermittent fasting on health markers in those with type 2 diabetes: A pilot study. Retrieved from https://www.ncbi.nlm.nih.gov/pubmed/28465792

Azevedo, F. R. de, Ikeoka, D., & Caramelli, B. (2013). Effects of intermittent fasting on metabolism in men. Retrieved from https://www.sciencedirect.com/science/article/pii/S0104423013000213

Barnosky, A. R., Hoddy, K. K., Unterman, T. G., & Varady, K. A. (2014). Intermittent fasting vs daily calorie restriction for type 2 diabetes prevention: a review of human findings. Retrieved from https://www.ncbi.nlm.nih.gov/pubmed/24993615

Barnosky, A. R., Hoddy, K. K., Unterman, T. G., & Varady, K. A. (2014). Intermittent fasting vs daily calorie restriction for type 2 diabetes prevention: a review of human findings. Retrieved from https://www.sciencedirect.com/science/article/pii/S193152441400200X

Bauersfeld, S. P., Kessler, C. S., Wischnewsky, M., Jaensch, A., Steckhan, N., Stange, R., ... Michalsen, A. (2018). The effects of short-term fasting on quality of life and tolerance to chemotherapy in patients with breast and ovarian cancer: a randomized cross-over pilot study. Retrieved from https://bmccancer.biomedcentral.com/articles/10.1186/s12885-018-4353-2

Baum, I. (2019). What Is the OMAD Diet? Everything You Need to Know About This Extreme Intermittent Fasting Weight-Loss Plan. Retrieved from https://www.health.com/weight-loss/omad-diet

Bendix, A. (2019). 8 signs your intermittent fasting diet has become unsafe or unhealthy. Retrieved from https://www.businessinsider.com/signs-intermittent-fasting-unsafe-unhealthy-2019-7

Berardi, J. (2015). Intermittent Fasting: Whos It For? (And, if Its Not for You, What to Do Instead). Retrieved from https://www.huffpost.com/entry/intermittent-fasting-whos_b_6236712

Biswas , C. (2020). The One Meal A Day Diet (OMAD Diet) – How It Works, Health Benefits, And Safety. Retrieved from https://www.stylecraze.com/articles/one-meal-a-day-diet-the-ultimate-guide/

Blindow, A. (2019). Fasting: the body's natural stem cell therapy. Retrieved from https://www.intelligent.life/blog/fast-bodys-natural-stem-cell-therapy

Brusie, C. (2017). Is Eating One Meal a Day a Safe and Effective Way to Lose Weight? Retrieved from https://www.healthline.com/health/one-meal-a-day

Carstensen, M. (2018). Intermittent Fasting Helps Reverse Type 2 Diabetes in 3 Men: Study: Everyday Health. Retrieved from https://www.everydayhealth.com/type-2-diabetes/diet/intermittent-fasting-helps-reverse-type-2-diabetes-men-study/

Carter, S., Clifton, P. M., & Keogh, J. B. (2018). Effect of Intermittent vs Continuous Energy Restricted Diet on Glycemic Control in Type 2 Diabetes. Retrieved from https://jamanetwork.com/journals/jamanetworkopen/fullarticle/2688344

Chaix, A., Zarrinpar, A., Miu, P., & Panda, S. (2014). Time-Restricted Feeding Is a Preventative and Therapeutic Intervention against Diverse Nutritional Challenges. Retrieved from https://www.sciencedirect.com/science/article/pii/S1550413114004987?via=ihub

Chander, R. (2018). I Tried Extreme Fasting by Eating Once a Day — Here's What Happened. Retrieved from https://www.healthline.com/health/food-nutrition/one-meal-a-day-diet#1

Cole, W. (2019). OMAD Is The Biggest New Diet Trend For Decreasing Inflammation & Increasing Longevity. Retrieved from https://www.mindbodygreen.com/articles/omad-diet-what-it-is-if-its-safe-and-how-to-do-it

Common Dos and Don'ts of eating One Meal a Day (OMAD) - Times of India. (2019). Retrieved from https://timesofindia.indiatimes.com/life-style/health-fitness/diet/common-dos-and-donts-of-eating-one-meal-a-day-omad/articleshow/70805234.cms

Cording, J. (2019). Is the Secret to Losing Weight More About When You Eat Than What? Retrieved from https://www.shape.com/healthy-eating/diet-tips/potential-intermittent-fasting-benefits-not-worth-dieting-risks

de Cabo, R., & Mattson, M. P. (2019). Effects of Intermittent Fasting on Health, Aging, and Disease. Retrieved from https://www.gwern.net/docs/longevity/2019-decabo.pdf

de Groot, S., Pijl, H., van der Hoeven, J. J. M., & Kroep, J. R. (2019). Effects of short-term fasting on cancer treatment. Retrieved from https://jeccr.biomedcentral.com/articles/10.1186/s13046-019-1189-9

DeSantis, S. (2019). 30 Minute Vegan Breakfast Burritos. Retrieved from https://www.veggiesdontbite.com/30-minute-vegan-breakfast-burritos-minimalist-baker-everyday-cooking/

Denton, M. (2019). Anti-Aging Benefits of Intermittent Fasting. Retrieved from https://neurohacker.com/anti-aging-benefits-of-intermittent-fasting

Descamps, O., Riondel, J., Ducros, V., & Roussel, A.-M. (2005). Mitochondrial production of reactive oxygen species and incidence of age-associated lymphoma in OF1 mice: effect of alternate-day fasting. Retrieved from https://www.ncbi.nlm.nih.gov/pubmed/16126250

Diet Review: Intermittent Fasting for Weight Loss. (2019). Retrieved from https://www.hsph.harvard.edu/nutritionsource/healthy-weight/diet-reviews/intermittent-fasting/

Duan, W., Guo, Z., Jiang, H., Ware, M., Li, X.-J., & Mattson, M. P. (2003). Dietary restriction normalizes glucose metabolism and BDNF levels, slows disease progression, and increases survival in huntingtin mutant mice. Retrieved from https://www.ncbi.nlm.nih.gov/pmc/articles/PMC151440/

Easy Full English Keto Breakfast: KetoDiet Blog. (2020). Retrieved from https://ketodietapp.com/Blog/lchf/easy-full-english-keto-breakfast

Easy Pork Chops With Asparagus and Hollandaise: KetoDiet Blog. (2020). Retrieved from https://ketodietapp.com/Blog/lchf/easy-pork-chops-with-asparagus-and-hollandaise

Effects of Intermittent Fasting on Health, Aging, and Disease. (2020). Retrieved from https://www.crossfit.com/essentials/effects-of-intermittent-fasting-on-health-aging-and-disease

Eldridge, L. (2019). Can Intermittent Fasting Help Treat or Prevent Cancer? Retrieved from https://www.verywellhealth.com/intermittent-fasting-and-cancer-4772239

Exton, L. (2020). Quick Keto Salmon Power Bowl: KetoDiet Blog. Retrieved from https://ketodietapp.com/Blog/lchf/quick-keto-salmon-power-bowl

Fessenden, M. (2015). Mostly the Old And Ill Ate Breakfast Until the Rise of the Working Man. Retrieved from https://www.smithsonianmag.com/smart-news/mostly-old-and-ill-ate-breakfast-until-rise-working-man-180954041/

Fletcher, J. (2020). One meal a day: Health benefits and risks. Retrieved from https://www.medicalnewstoday.com/articles/320125

Fung, J. (2016). How to Renew Your Body: Fasting and Autophagy. Retrieved from https://www.dietdoctor.com/renew-body-fasting-autophagy

Furmli, S., Elmasry, R., Ramos, M., & Fung, J. (2017). Therapeutic use of intermittent fasting for people with type 2 diabetes as an alternative to insulin. Retrieved from https://casereports.bmj.com/content/2018/bcr-2017-221854.full

Gleeson, J. R. (2019). Intermittent Fasting: Is it Right for You? Retrieved from https://healthblog.uofmhealth.org/wellness-prevention/intermittent-fasting-it-right-for-you

Gleeson, J. R. (2019). Intermittent Fasting: Is it Right for You? Retrieved from https://healthblog.uofmhealth.org/wellness-prevention/intermittent-fasting-it-right-for-you

Goodrick, Charles L., I., K., D., A., M., Freeman, R., J., ... Reynolds. (1983). Differential Effects of Intermittent Feeding and Voluntary Exercise on Body Weight and Lifespan in Adult Rats 1. Retrieved from https://academic.oup.com/geronj/article-abstract/38/1/36/570019

Gunnars, K. (2020). 6 Popular Ways to Do Intermittent Fasting. Retrieved from https://www.healthline.com/nutrition/6-ways-to-do-intermittent-fasting

Gunnars, K. (2017). How Intermittent Fasting Can Help You Lose Weight. Retrieved from https://www.healthline.com/nutrition/intermittent-fasting-and-weight-loss

Gunnars, K. (2016). 10 Evidence-Based Health Benefits of Intermittent Fasting. Retrieved from https://www.healthline.com/nutrition/10-health-benefits-of-intermittent-fasting

Haridy, R. (2019). Review of intermittent fasting research suggests broad health benefits. Retrieved from https://newatlas.

com/health-wellbeing/review-intermittent-fasting-research-health-benefits-johns-hopkins/

Hine, C., Harputlugil, E., Zhang, Y., Ruckenstuhl, C., Cheon Lee, B., Brace, L., ... Mitchell, J. R. (2014). Endogenous Hydrogen Sulfide Production Is Essential for Dietary Restriction Benefits. Retrieved from https://www.cell.com/cell/fulltext/S0092-8674(14)01525-6

How to start OMAD - One Meal a Day. (2018). Retrieved from https://desireepeeples.com/start-omad-one-meal-day/

Intermittent Fasting: 4 Different Types Explained. (2019). Retrieved from https://health.clevelandclinic.org/intermittent-fasting-4-different-types-explained/

Jarreau, P. B. (2018). Eating (Or rather, Fasting) Our Way to Rejuvenated Stem Cells? Retrieved from https://medium.com/lifeomic/eating-or-rather-fasting-our-way-to-rejuvenated-stem-cells-e4302a49e597

Johnson, J. B., Summer, W., Cutler, R. G., Martin, B., Hyun, D.-H., Dixit, V. D., ... Mattson, M. P. (2007). Alternate day calorie restriction improves clinical findings and reduces markers of oxidative stress and inflammation in overweight adults with moderate asthma. Retrieved from https://www.ncbi.nlm.nih.gov/pubmed/17291990/

Johnstone, A. (2015). Fasting for weight loss: an effective strategy or latest dieting trend? Retrieved from https://www.

ncbi.nlm.nih.gov/pubmed/25540982

Jordan, S., Tung, N., Casanova-Acebes, M., Chang, C., Cantoni, C., Zhang, D., ... Merad, M. (2019). Dietary Intake Regulates the Circulating Inflammatory Monocyte Pool. Retrieved from https://www.cell.com/cell/fulltext/S0092-8674(19)30850-5

Kerndt, P. R., Naughton, J. L., Driscoll, C. E., & Loxterkamp, D. A. (1982). Fasting: the history, pathophysiology and complications. Retrieved from https://www.ncbi.nlm.nih.gov/pubmed/6758355

Landsverk, G. (2019). Intermittent fasting may help slow aging and diseases like cancer and diabetes - even if you don't lose weight. Retrieved from https://www.insider.com/intermittent-fasting-slows-aging-cancer-diabetes-heart-disease-study-2019-12

Lee, C., Raffaghello, L., Brandhorst, S., Safdie, F. M., Bianchi, G., Martin-Montalvo, A., ... Longo, V. D. (2012). Fasting cycles retard growth of tumors and sensitize a range of cancer cell types to chemotherapy. Retrieved from https://www.ncbi.nlm.nih.gov/pubmed/22323820

Lee, J., Duan, W., Long, J. M., Ingram, D. K., & Mattson, M. P. (2000). Dietary restriction increases the number of newly generated neural cells, and induces BDNF expression, in the dentate gyrus of rats. Retrieved from https://www.ncbi.nlm.nih.gov/pubmed/11220789

Leech, J. (2019). 5 Stats That Show Why Intermittent Fasting is Powerful for Weight Loss. Retrieved from https://www.dietvsdisease.org/intermittent-fasting-is-powerful-for-weight-loss/

Leonard, J. (2020). 7 formas de hacer ayuno intermitente: Los mejores métodos. Retrieved from https://www.medicalnewstoday.com/articles/322293

Levy, J. (2018). Benefits of Autophagy, Plus How to Induce It. Retrieved from https://draxe.com/health/benefits-of-autophagy/

Li, L., Wang, Z., & Zuo, Z. (2013). Chronic intermittent fasting improves cognitive functions and brain structures in mice. Retrieved from https://www.ncbi.nlm.nih.gov/pmc/articles/PMC3670843/

Lindberg, S. (2018). Autophagy: What You Need to Know. Retrieved from https://www.healthline.com/health/autophagy

London, J. (2019, May 28). The Trendy OMAD Diet Has a Ton of Potentially Scary Side Effects. Retrieved from https://www.goodhousekeeping.com/health/diet-nutrition/a27506052/omad-diet/

Low-Carb Steak Taco Bowl: KetoDiet Blog. (2020). Retrieved from https://ketodietapp.com/Blog/lchf/low-carb-steak-taco-bowl

Magyar, O. (2017). Intermittent Fasting For Better Brain Health? Retrieved from https://neurotrition.ca/blog/intermittent-fasting-better-brain-health

Marosi, K., Moehl , K., Navas-Enamorado, I., Mitchell, S. J., Zhang, Y., Lehrmann , E., ... Mattson, M. P. (2018). Metabolic and molecular framework for the enhancement of endurance by intermittent food deprivation. Retrieved from https://www.fasebj.org/doi/10.1096/fj.201701378RR

Mattson, M. P., Moehl, K., Ghena, N., Schmaedick, M., & Cheng, A. (2018). Intermittent metabolic switching, neuroplasticity and brain health. Retrieved from https://www.ncbi.nlm.nih.gov/pubmed/29321682

Mattson, M. P. (2005). Energy intake, meal frequency, and health: a neurobiological perspective. Retrieved from https://www.ncbi.nlm.nih.gov/pubmed/16011467

McLeod, C. (2019). Intermittent fasting is trendy but dietitians warn against it. Retrieved from https://www.bodyandsoul.com.au/nutrition/nutrition-tips/the-6-people-who-shouldnt-try-intermittent-fasting-according-to-a-dietitian/news-story/ca97f74fc904811f4b78281824dea72c

Migala, J. (2020). 7 Types of Intermittent Fasting: Which Is Best for You?: Everyday Health. Retrieved from https://www.everydayhealth.com/diet-nutrition/diet/types-intermittent-fasting-which-best-you/

Mihaylova, M. M., Cheng, C.-W., Cao, A. Q., Tripathi, S., Mana, M. D., Bauer-Rowe, K. E., ... Yilmaz, Ö. H. (2018). Fasting Activates Fatty Acid Oxidation to Enhance Intestinal Stem Cell Function during Homeostasis and Aging. Retrieved from https://www.sciencedirect.com/science/article/pii/S1934590918301632

Moller, N., Vendelbo, M. H., Kampmann, U., Christensen, B., Madsen, M., Norrelund, H., & Jorgensen, J. O. (2009). Growth hormone and protein metabolism. Retrieved from https://www.ncbi.nlm.nih.gov/pubmed/19773097

Moro, T., Tinsley, G., Bianco, A., Marcolin, G., Pacelli, Q. F., Battaglia, G., ... Paoli, A. (2016). Effects of eight weeks of time-restricted feeding (16/8) on basal metabolism, maximal strength, body composition, inflammation, and cardiovascular risk factors in resistance-trained males. Retrieved from https://translational-medicine.biomedcentral.com/articles/10.1186/s12967-016-1044-0

Nørrelund, H., Nair, K. S., Jørgensen, J. O., Christiansen, J. S., & Møller, N. (2001). The protein-retaining effects of growth hormone during fasting involve inhibition of muscle-protein breakdown. Retrieved from https://www.ncbi.nlm.nih.gov/pubmed/11147801

O'Flanagan, C. H., Smith, L. A., McDonell, S. B., & Hursting, S. D. (2017). When less may be more: calorie restriction and response to cancer therapy. Retrieved from https://www.ncbi.nlm.nih.gov/pubmed/28539118

OMAD DIET: THE ULTIMATE GUIDE. (2019). Retrieved from https://omadmealplan.com/

Oppenheim, S. (2019). Is Intermittent Fasting Really The Healthiest Way To Eat? Not For Everyone. Retrieved from https://www.forbes.com/sites/serenaoppenheim/2019/01/24/is-intermittent-fasting-really-the-healthiest-way-to-eat-not-for-everyone/#276fd2d13606

Paddock, C. (2018). How fasting boosts exercise's effects on endurance. Retrieved from https://www.medicalnewstoday.com/articles/321056

Park, M. (2010). Nearing 50, Renaissance jock Herschel Walker breaks fitness rules. Retrieved from http://edition.cnn.com/2010/HEALTH/10/11/herschel.fitness.martial.arts/index.html

Pattillo, A. (2019). The Truth Behind What Intermittent Fasting Does to Your Body. Retrieved from https://www.inverse.com/article/57625-what-intermittent-fasting-actually-does-to-your-body

Pawlowski, A. (2019). What is the OMAD diet? Learn how the one-meal-a-day plan works. Retrieved from https://www.today.com/health/what-omad-diet-learn-how-one-meal-day-diet-works-t146204

Permanente, K. (n.d.). How our bodies turn food into energy. Retrieved from https://wa.kaiserpermanente.org/healthAndWellness?item=/common/healthAndWellness/conditions/diabetes/foodProcess.html

Pleimling, A. (2017). Trendy or troublesome? Get the facts on intermittent fasting. Retrieved from https://www.allinahealth.org/healthysetgo/nourish/trendy-or-troublesome-the-facts-on-intermittent-fasting

Phillips, M. C. L. (2019). Fasting as a Therapy in Neurological Disease. Retrieved from https://www.ncbi.nlm.nih.gov/pmc/articles/PMC6836141/

Presto, G. (2017). Is Intermittent Fasting Right For You? Retrieved from https://www.bornfitness.com/intermittent-fasting/

Research on intermittent fasting shows health benefits. (2020, February 27). Retrieved from https://www.nia.nih.gov/news/research-intermittent-fasting-shows-health-benefits

Researchers discover that fasting reduces inflammation and improves chronic inflammatory diseases. (2019). Retrieved from https://medicalxpress.com/news/2019-08-fasting-inflammation-chronic-inflammatory-diseases.html

Ries, J. (2020). This Is Your Body On Intermittent Fasting. Retrieved from https://www.huffpost.com/entry/body-intermittent-fasting_l_5e0a3220c5b6b5a713b22dcb?

guccounter=1&guce_referrer=
aHR0cHM6Ly93d3cuZ29vZ2xlLmNvbS8&guce_referrer_sig=
AQAAAC-
HM3NWPXeuZI89BsKO_6IpI8l9andTLuWwBQJfgG-
AsuIWgujK_56SnSe6nwtztpxQJ50POffVrpAasbAvte9Zq5Z31
m4DPBrmQfjl-gS1ahKuyRQNZApPT-
6VAiMjRY5SqN1g6Vcfx_jg2BiwVYsMz8SklicgTXv6h1SZI-GS

Rinzler, C. A., & DeVault, K. (n.d.). The Human Digestion Process (or, What Happens after You Eat Food). Retrieved from https://www.dummies.com/education/science/biology/the-human-digestion-process-or-what-happens-after-you-eat-food/

Rose, E. (2020). OMAD: What is One Meal a Day Fasting, and Should You Try It? Retrieved from https://www.bulletproof.com/diet/intermittent-fasting/omad-one-meal-a-day-diet/

Rumi Quote: "Fasting is the first principle of medicine; fast and see the strength of the spirit reveal itself.". (n.d.). Retrieved from https://quotefancy.com/quote/904488/Rumi-Fasting-is-the-first-principle-of-medicine-fast-and-see-the-strength-of-the-spirit

Save, K. (2019). What really happens to your body during intermittent fasting. Retrieved from https://www.bodyandsoul.com.au/diet/diets/what-really-happens-to-your-body-during-intermittent-fasting/news-story/92cdbf27507d9fa3afe30eaab3172b5e

Scher, B. (2020). What You Need to Know About OMAD. Retrieved from https://www.dietdoctor.com/intermittent-fasting/omad

Schmidt, M. (2020). What Science Says About the Weight-Loss Potential of 'OMAD' Fasting - The One-Meal-a-Day Diet. Retrieved from https://www.discovermagazine.com/health/what-science-says-about-the-weight-loss-potential-of-omad-fasting-the-one

Seimon, R. V., Roekenes, J. A., Zibellini, J., Zhu, B., Gibson, A. A., Hills, A. P., ... Sainsbury, A. (2015). Do intermittent diets provide physiological benefits over continuous diets for weight loss? A systematic review of clinical trials. Retrieved from https://www.sciencedirect.com/science/article/abs/pii/S0303720715300800?via=ihub

Sigurdsson, A. F. (2020). Intermittent Fasting and Health – The Scientific Evidence. Retrieved from https://www.docsopinion.com/intermittent-fasting

Sisson, M. (2020). 7 Tips and Considerations for Eating One Meal a Day. Retrieved from https://www.marksdailyapple.com/7-tips-and-considerations-for-eating-one-meal-a-day/

Sogawa, H., & Kubo, C. (2000). Influence of short-term repeated fasting on the longevity of female (NZB×NZW)F1 mice. Retrieved from https://www.sciencedirect.com/science/article/abs/pii/S0047637400001093

Southard, L. (2020). What is OMAD diet: Why eating one meal a day isn't recommended by experts. Retrieved from https://www.insider.com/what-is-omad-diet

Stieg, C. (2019). Is The OMAD Diet The New Intermittent Fasting? Retrieved from https://www.refinery29.com/en-us/eating-one-meal-a-day-diet-trend

Stote, K. S., Baer, D. J., Spears, K., Paul, D. R., Harris, G. K., Rumpler, W. V., ... Mattson, M. P. (2007). A controlled trial of reduced meal frequency without caloric restriction in healthy, normal-weight, middle-aged adults. Retrieved from https://www.ncbi.nlm.nih.gov/pmc/articles/PMC2645638/

Sweet Potato Taco Bowl. (2019). Retrieved from https://www.mykitchenlove.com/sweet-potato-taco-bowl/

Tello, M. (2020). Intermittent fasting: Surprising update. Retrieved from https://www.health.harvard.edu/blog/intermittent-fasting-surprising-update-2018062914156

Templeman, I., Gonzalez, J. T., Thompson, D., & Betts, J. A. (2020). The role of intermittent fasting and meal timing in weight management and metabolic health. Retrieved from https://www.ncbi.nlm.nih.gov/pubmed/31023390

Templeton, L. (2019). Intermittent fasting can help ease metabolic syndrome. Retrieved from https://www.medicalnewstoday.com/articles/327247

The Dangers of Intermittent Fasting. (2019). Retrieved from https://centerfordiscovery.com/blog/the-dangers-of-intermittent-fasting/

The OMAD Diet: Is Having One Meal A Day Effective? (2020). Retrieved from https://betterme.world/articles/omad-diet/

The Warrior Diet: Review and Beginner's Guide. (2018). Retrieved from https://www.healthline.com/nutrition/warrior-diet-guide

Tinsley, G. M., & La Bounty, P. M. (2015). Effects of intermittent fasting on body composition and clinical health markers in humans. Retrieved from https://academic.oup.com/nutritionreviews/article/73/10/661/1849182

Top 10 Tips for OMAD - Tips for One Meal a Day Diet. (2019). Retrieved from http://siimland.com/top-10-tips-for-omad-tips-for-one-meal-a-day-diet/

Varady, K. A., & Hellerstein, M. K. (2007). Alternate-day fasting and chronic disease prevention: a review of human and animal trials. Retrieved from https://www.ncbi.nlm.nih.gov/pubmed/17616757?dopt=Abstract

Varady, K. A., Bhutani, S., Church, E. C., & Klempel, M. C. (2009). Short-term modified alternate-day fasting: a novel dietary strategy for weight loss and cardioprotection in obese adults. Retrieved from https://www.ncbi.nlm.nih.gov/pubmed/19793855

Varady, K. A. (2011). Intermittent versus daily calorie restriction: which diet regimen is more effective for weight loss? Retrieved from https://www.ncbi.nlm.nih.gov/pubmed/21410865

Weindruch, R., & Sohal, R. S. (1997). Seminars in medicine of the Beth Israel Deaconess Medical Center. Caloric intake and aging. Retrieved from https://www.ncbi.nlm.nih.gov/pmc/articles/PMC2851235/

West, H. (2016). Does Intermittent Fasting Boost Your Metabolism? Retrieved from https://www.healthline.com/nutrition/intermittent-fasting-metabolism

What happens to the food we eat? - (Food and Body Function). (n.d.). Retrieved from http://apjcn.nhri.org.tw/server/info/books-phds/books/foodfacts/html/maintext/main3a.html

Wilkinson, M. J., Manoogian, E. N. C., Zadourian, A., Navlakha, S., Lo, H., Fakhouri, S., … Taub, P. R. (2019). Ten-Hour Time-Restricted Eating Reduces Weight, Blood Pressure, and Atherogenic Lipids in Patients with Metabolic Syndrome. Retrieved from https://www.cell.com/cell-metabolism/fulltext/S1550-4131(19)30611-4

Zahid, U. (2019). (Ultimate Guide) All You Need to Know About OMAD Diet. Retrieved from https://ashrafchaudhryblog.com/omad-diet/

Zarrinpar, A., Chaix, A., Yooseph, S., & Panda, S. (2014). Diet and feeding pattern affect the diurnal dynamics of the gut microbiome. Retrieved from https://www.ncbi.nlm.nih.gov/pubmed/25470548

Zhang, J., Zhan, Z., Li, X., Xing, A., Jiang, C., Chen, Y., ... An, L. (2017). Intermittent Fasting Protects against Alzheimer's Disease Possible through Restoring Aquaporin-4 Polarity. Retrieved from https://www.ncbi.nlm.nih.gov/pmc/articles/PMC5712566/

Made in the USA
Monee, IL
23 September 2020